# Advanced PAP Therapies and Non-invasive Ventilation

*Editors*

LEE K. BROWN
SHAHROKH JAVAHERI

# SLEEP MEDICINE CLINICS

www.sleep.theclinics.com

*Consulting Editor*
TEOFILO LEE-CHIONG Jr

December 2017 • Volume 12 • Number 4

**ELSEVIER**

1600 John F. Kennedy Boulevard • Suite 1800 • Philadelphia, Pennsylvania, 19103-2899

http://www.theclinics.com

**SLEEP MEDICINE CLINICS Volume 12, Number 4**
**December 2017, ISSN 1556-407X, ISBN-13: 978-0-323-55298-1**

Editor: Colleen Dietzler
Developmental Editor: Donald Mumford

**Photocopying**
Single photocopies of single articles may be made for personal use as allowed by national copyright laws. Permission of the Publisher and payment of a fee is required for all other photocopying, including multiple or systematic copying, copying for advertising or promotional purposes, resale, and all forms of document delivery. Special rates are available for educational institutions that wish to make photocopies for non-profit educational classroom use. For information on how to seek permission visit www.elsevier.com/permissions or call: (+44) 1865 843830 (UK)/(+1) 215 239 3804 (USA).

**Derivative Works**
Subscribers may reproduce tables of contents or prepare lists of articles including abstracts for internal circulation within their institutions. Permission of the Publisher is required for resale or distribution outside the institution. Permission of the Publisher is required for all other derivative works, including compilations and translations (please consult www.elsevier.com/permissions).

**Electronic Storage or Usage**
Permission of the Publisher is required to store or use electronically any material contained in this periodical, including any article or part of an article (please consult www.elsevier.com/permissions). Except as outlined above, no part of this publication may be reproduced, stored in a retrieval system or transmitted in any form or by any means, electronic, mechanical, photocopying, recording or otherwise, without prior written permission of the Publisher.

**Notice**
No responsibility is assumed by the Publisher for any injury and/or damage to persons or property as a matter of products liability, negligence or otherwise, or from any use or operation of any methods, products, instructions or ideas contained in the material herein. Because of rapid advances in the medical sciences, in particular, independent verification of diagnoses and drug dosages should be made. Although all advertising material is expected to conform to ethical (medical) standards, inclusion in this publication does not constitute a guarantee or endorsement of the quality or value of such product or of the claims made of it by its manufacturer.

*Sleep Medicine Clinics* (ISSN 1556-407X) is published quarterly by Elsevier Inc., 360 Park Avenue South, New York, NY 10010-1710. Months of issue are March, June, September and December. Business and Editorial Offices: 1600 John F. Kennedy Blvd., Ste. 1800, Philadelphia, PA 19103-2899. Customer Service Office: 3251 Riverport Lane, Maryland Heights, MO 63043. Periodicals postage paid at New York, NY and additional mailing offices. Subscription prices are $203.00 per year (US individuals), $100.00 (US students), $476.00 (US institutions), $244.00 (Canadian and international individuals), $135.00 (Canadian and international students), $540.00 (Canadian institutions) and $529.00 (International institutions). Foreign air speed delivery is included in all *Clinics* subscription prices. All prices are subject to change without notice. **POSTMASTER:** Send change of address to *Sleep Medicine Clinics*, Elsevier Health Sciences Division, Subscription Customer Service, 3251 Riverport Lane, Maryland Heights, MO 63043. Customer Service: **Tel: 1-800-654-2452 (U.S. and Canada); 314-447-8871 (outside U.S. and Canada). Fax: 314-447-8029. E-mail: journalscustomerservice-usa@elsevier.com (for print support); journalsonline support-usa@elsevier.com (for online support).**

*Reprints.* For copies of 100 or more of articles in this publication, please contact the Commercial Reprints Department, Elsevier Inc., 360 Park Avenue South, New York, NY 10010-1710. Tel.: 212-633-3874; Fax: 212-633-3820; E-mail: reprints@elsevier.com.

*Sleep Medicine Clinics* is covered in *MEDLINE/PubMed (Index Medicus)*.

## PROGRAM OBJECTIVE
The goal of *Sleep Clinics of North America* is to keep practicing physicians up to date with current clinical practice by providing timely articles reviewing the state of the art in patient care.

## TARGET AUDIENCE
All practicing physicians and other healthcare professionals.

## LEARNING OBJECTIVES
Upon completion of this activity, participants will be able to:
1. Review current and emerging technologies in positive airway pressure devices.
2. Discuss emerging treatments for obstructive sleep apnea.
3. Recognize current and future applications of airway pressure technology.

## ACCREDITATION
The Elsevier Office of Continuing Medical Education (EOCME) is accredited by the Accreditation Council for Continuing Medical Education (ACCME) to provide continuing medical education for physicians.

The EOCME designates this enduring material for a maximum of 15 *AMA PRA Category 1 Credit*(s)™. Physicians should claim only the credit commensurate with the extent of their participation in the activity.

All other healthcare professionals requesting continuing education credit for this enduring material will be issued a certificate of participation.

## DISCLOSURE OF CONFLICTS OF INTEREST
The EOCME assesses conflict of interest with its instructors, faculty, planners, and other individuals who are in a position to control the content of CME activities. All relevant conflicts of interest that are identified are thoroughly vetted by EOCME for fair balance, scientific objectivity, and patient care recommendations. EOCME is committed to providing its learners with CME activities that promote improvements or quality in healthcare and not a specific proprietary business or a commercial interest.

**The planning committee, staff, authors and editors listed below have identified no financial relationships or relationships to products or devices they or their spouse/life partner have with commercial interest related to the content of this CME activity:**

John R. Bach, MD; Ahmed S. BaHammam, MD, FACP; Maly Oron Benhamou, MD; Susmita Chowdhuri, MD, MS; Jacob F. Collen, MD; Claire Colas Des Francs, MD; Marie Nguyen Dibra, MD; Colleen Dietzler; Pierre Escorrou, MD, PhD; Antonio M. Esquinas, MD, PhD, FCCP; Anjali Fortna; Neil Freedman, MD; Shahrokh Javaheri, MD; Karin G. Johnson, MD; Christopher J. Lettieri, MD; Leah Logan; Bushra Mina, MD; Amélie Sagniez, MSc; Rajakumar Venkatesan; Mary H. Wagner, MD; Kaixian Zhu, PhD.

**The planning committee, staff, authors and editors listed below have identified financial relationships or relationships to products or devices they or their spouse/life partner have with commercial interest related to *the content of this CME activity*:**

**Richard Barnett Berry, MD** has research support from Koninklijke Philips N.V. and NightBalance B.V.
**Lee K. Brown, MD** is a consultant/advisor for Considine and Associates and Koninklijke Philips N.V, has an employment affiliation with Current Opinion in Pulmonary Medicine, and receives royalties/patents from Wolters Kluwer.
**Alastair J. Glossop, MD** is on the speakers' bureau for, a consultant/advisor for, and receives royalties/patents from Armstrong Medical.
**Teofilo Lee-Chiong Jr, MD** is a consultant/advisor for Elsevier and CareCore National, has stock ownsership in and an employment affiliation with Elsevier, and receieves royalties/patents from Lippincott; Oxford University Press; CreateSpace, a DBA of On-Demand Publishing, LLC.; and John Wiley & Sons, Inc.
**Amanda J. Piper, PhD** is on the speakers' bureau for ResMed and Asia Pacific, and is a consultant/advisor for Koninklijke Philips N.V.
**David M. Rapoport, MD** is a consultant/advisor for Fisher & Paykel Healthcare Limited and Eight, Inc, has stock ownership in Eight, Inc, and has research support from Fisher and Paykel Healthcare Limited.
**Emerson M. Wickwire, PhD** is a consultant/advisor for Merck & Co., Inc, has stock ownership in WellTap, and has research support from American Academy of Sleep Medicine; Merck & Co., Inc; and ResMed.
**Scott G. Williams, MD** is a consultant/advisor for the American Academy of Sleep Medicine.

## UNAPPROVED/OFF-LABEL USE DISCLOSURE
The EOCME requires CME faculty to disclose to the participants:
1. When products or procedures being discussed are off-label, unlabelled, experimental, and/or investigational (not US Food and Drug Administration [FDA] approved); and
2. Any limitations on the information presented, such as data that are preliminary or that represent ongoing research, interim analyses, and/or unsupported opinions. Faculty may discuss information about pharmaceutical agents that is outside of

FDA-approved labelling. This information is intended solely for CME and is not intended to promote off-label use of these medications. If you have any questions, contact the medical affairs department of the manufacturer for the most recent prescribing information.

## TO ENROLL
To enroll in the Sleep Medicines Clinic Continuing Medical Education program, call customer service at 1-800-654-2452 or sign up online at http://www.theclinics.com/home/cme. The CME program is available to subscribers for an additional annual fee of USD $140.

## METHOD OF PARTICIPATION
In order to claim credit, participants must complete the following:
1. Complete enrolment as indicated above.
2. Read the activity.
3. Complete the CME Test and Evaluation. Participants must achieve a score of 70% on the test. All CME Tests and Evaluations must be completed online.

## CME INQUIRIES/SPECIAL NEEDS
For all CME inquiries or special needs, please contact elsevierCME@elsevier.com.

# SLEEP MEDICINE CLINICS

**THE CLINICS ARE AVAILABLE ONLINE!**
Access your subscription at:
www.theclinics.com

# Contributors

## CONSULTING EDITOR

**TEOFILO LEE-CHIONG Jr, MD**
Professor of Medicine, National Jewish Health,
Professor of Medicine, University of Colorado,
Denver, Colorado, USA; Chief Medical Liaison,
Philips Respironics, Pennsylvania, USA

## EDITORS

**LEE K. BROWN, MD**
Professor of Internal Medicine and Pediatrics
and Senior Vice Chair, Clinical Affairs,
Department of Internal Medicine, The
University of New Mexico School of Medicine,
Professor, Department of Electrical and
Computer Engineering, The University of New
Mexico School of Engineering, Medical
Director, The University of New Mexico Health
System Sleep Disorders Centers,
Albuquerque, New Mexico, USA

**SHAHROKH JAVAHERI, MD**
Professor Emeritus, University of Cincinnati,
Medical Director, Montgomery Sleep
Laboratory, TriHealth Sleep Center, Pulmonary
and Sleep Division, Bethesda North Hospital;
Adjunct Professor, Division of Cardiology,
Department of Internal Medicine, The Ohio
State University College of Medicine,
Columbus, Ohio, USA

## AUTHORS

**JOHN R. BACH, MD**
Professor of Physical Medicine and
Rehabilitation, and Neurology, Department
of Physical Medicine and Rehabilitation,
Rutgers New Jersey Medical School, Medical
Director, Center for Noninvasive Mechanical
Ventilation Alternatives and Pulmonary
Rehabilitation, University Hospital, Newark,
New Jersey, USA

**AHMED S. BaHAMMAM, MD, FACP**
Director, University Sleep Disorders
Center, Department of Medicine, College of
Medicine, National Plan for Science and
Technology, King Saud University, Riyadh,
Saudi Arabia

**MALY ORON BENHAMOU, MD**
Department of Medicine, Division of Pulmonary
and Critical Care Medicine, Northwell Health,
Lenox Hill Hospital, New York, New York, USA

**RICHARD BARNETT BERRY, MD**
Professor of Medicine, Medical Director of
the UF Health Sleep Disorders Center,
University of Florida Sleep Medicine
Fellowship Director, Department of
Sleep Medicine, UF Health Sleep Center,
University of Florida, Gainesville, Florida,
USA

**LEE K. BROWN, MD**
Professor of Internal Medicine and Pediatrics
and Senior Vice Chair, Clinical Affairs,
Department of Internal Medicine, The
University of New Mexico School of Medicine,
Professor, Department of Electrical and
Computer Engineering, The University of
New Mexico School of Engineering, Medical
Director, The University of New Mexico Health
System Sleep Disorders Centers,
Albuquerque, New Mexico, USA

**SUSMITA CHOWDHURI, MD, MS**
Associate Professor of Medicine, Sleep
Medicine Section, John D. Dingell VA Medical
Center, Wayne State University, Detroit,
Michigan, USA

**JACOB F. COLLEN, MD**
Assistant Professor of Medicine,
Program Director, Sleep Medicine
Fellowship, Department of Pulmonary, Critical
Care, and Sleep Medicine, Walter Reed
National Military Medical Center, Bethesda,
Maryland, USA

**CLAIRE COLAS DES FRANCS, MD**
Sleep Disorders Center, AP-HP Antoine-
Béclère Hospital, Clamart, France

**MARIE NGUYEN DIBRA, MD**
Clinical Assistant Professor, Division of
Pulmonary, Critical Care, and Sleep Medicine,
Department of Sleep Medicine, UF Health
Sleep Center, University of Florida, Gainesville,
Florida, USA

**PIERRE ESCOURROU, MD, PhD**
Sleep Disorders Center, AP-HP Antoine-
Béclère Hospital, Clamart, France

**ANTONIO M. ESQUINAS, MD, PhD, FCCP**
Intensive Care and Non-invasive Ventilatory
Unit, Hospital Morales Meseguer, Murcia,
Spain

**NEIL FREEDMAN, MD**
Division Head, Pulmonary, Critical Care,
Allergy and Immunology, Department
of Medicine, NorthShore University
HealthSystem, Evanston, Illinois, USA

**ALASTAIR J. GLOSSOP, MD**
Department of Critical Care, Sheffield Teaching
Hospitals NHS Foundation Trust, Royal
Hallamshire Hospital, Sheffield, United
Kingdom

**SHAHROKH JAVAHERI, MD**
Professor Emeritus, University of Cincinnati,
Medical Director, Montgomery Sleep
Laboratory, TriHealth Sleep Center, Pulmonary
and Sleep Division, Bethesda North Hospital;

Adjunct Professor, Division of Cardiology,
Department of Internal Medicine, The Ohio
State University College of Medicine,
Columbus, Ohio, USA

**KARIN G. JOHNSON, MD**
Assistant Professor of Neurology and Vice
Chair, Department of Neurology, University of
Massachusetts Medical School, Baystate,
Neurodiagnostics and Sleep Center, Baystate
Medical Center, Springfield, Massachusetts,
USA

**CHRISTOPHER J. LETTIERI, MD**
Professor of Medicine, Department of
Pulmonary, Critical Care, and Sleep Medicine,
Walter Reed National Military Medical Center,
Bethesda, Maryland, USA

**BUSHRA MINA, MD**
Department of Medicine, Division of
Pulmonary and Critical Care Medicine,
Northwell Health, Lenox Hill Hospital, New
York, New York, USA

**AMANDA J. PIPER, PhD**
Department of Respiratory and Sleep
Medicine, Royal Prince Alfred Hospital,
Camperdown, New South Wales, Australia;
Associate Professor, Central Medical School -
Central, The University of Sydney, Sydney,
New South Wales, Australia

**DAVID M. RAPOPORT, MD**
Division of Pulmonary, Critical Care and Sleep
Medicine, Icahn School of Medicine at Mount
Sinai, New York, New York, USA

**AMÉLIE SAGNIEZ, MSc**
Centre Explor, Air Liquide Healthcare, Gentilly,
France

**MARY H. WAGNER, MD**
Associate Professor of Pediatric
Pulmonology, University of Florida Sleep
Medicine Fellowship Co-Director, Department
of Sleep Medicine, Director of the Pediatric
Sleep Laboratory, UF Health Sleep Disorders
Center, UF Health Sleep Center, Gainesville,
Florida, USA

**EMERSON M. WICKWIRE, PhD**
Assistant Professor and Director,
Insomnia Program, Department of Psychiatry,
Sleep Disorders Center, Division of
Pulmonary and Critical Care Medicine,
Department of Medicine, University of
Maryland School of Medicine, Baltimore,
Maryland, USA

**SCOTT G. WILLIAMS, MD**
Associate Professor of Medicine, Chief of
Sleep Medicine, Department of Pulmonary,
Critical Care, and Sleep Medicine, Walter Reed
National Military Medical Center, Bethesda,
Maryland, USA

**KAIXIAN ZHU, PhD**
Centre Explor, Air Liquide Healthcare, Gentilly,
France

# Contents

Since the introduction of continuous positive airway pressure (PAP) for the treatment of obstructive sleep apnea (OSA) in 1981, PAP technology has diversified exponentially. Compact and quiet fixed continuous PAP flow generators, autotitrating PAP devices, and bilevel PAP devices that can treat multiple sleep-disordered breathing phenotypes, including OSA, central sleep apnea (CSA), combinations of OSA and CSA, and hypoventilation, are available. Adaptive servoventilators can suppress Hunter-Cheyne-Stokes breathing and CSA and treat coexisting obstructive events. Volume-assured pressure support PAP apparatus purports to provide a targeted degree of ventilatory assistance while also treating cooccurring OSA and/or CSA.

Positive airway pressure (PAP) devices use different proprietary algorithms for sleep-disordered breathing event detection and response. Most device evaluations are based on clinical studies, which have obvious limitations. As a complementary approach, bench studies provide an analysis of algorithms in predefined conditions, which allows understanding contradictory results observed in clinical studies. But such studies cannot provide long-term treatment data and physiologic effects of treatment. It is important to understand the advantages and the limitations of both kinds of studies. Combining results of bench tests and clinical studies is essential to improve the management of patients with PAP treatment.

Positive airway pressure (PAP) remains the primary therapy for most patients with obstructive sleep apnea (OSA). CPAP, APAP, and BPAP are all reasonable therapies that can be used for patients with uncomplicated OSA across the spectrum of disease severity. BPAP should be considered for patients who are nonadherent to CPAP or APAP therapy because of pressure intolerance. Several additional factors should be considered when choosing the type of PAP device for a given patient, including associated symptoms and comorbid medical problems, cost, access to online data management and patient portals, and the portability for the device for patients who travel frequently.

Patient interface preference is a key factor in positive airway pressure compliance. Local side effects are common. Proper mask fitting and patient education are important. Masks should seal well and fit comfortably. Nasal, nasal pillow, and oronasal masks can be effective interfaces. Most patients with obstructive sleep apnea prefer a nasal mask. Oronasal masks can be a useful alternative. Nasal pillows can reduce mask size and improve comfort. Oronasal masks may require a higher pressure. A significantly lower pressure may be effective with a nasal interface. Proper mask fitting requires testing the mask seal under the treatment pressure.

Obstructive sleep apnea is a common and treatable condition, but therapeutic adherence is limited by numerous factors. Despite advances in positive airway pressure (PAP) technology and a multitude of effective pharmacologic and behavioral therapeutic interventions to overcome the most common barriers to PAP, adherence has not increased significantly over the past 30 years. This article aims to identify the most important factors that affect adherence, common barriers to treatment, and evidence-based treatment strategies to maximize the effectiveness of PAP treatment. Complications of PAP treatment and mitigation techniques are also discussed.

Central sleep apnea (CSA) and Hunter-Cheyne-Stokes breathing (HCSB) are caused by failure of the pontomedullary pacemaker generating breathing rhythm. CSA/HCSB may complicate several disorders causing recurrent arousals and desaturations. Common causes of CSA in adults are congestive heart failure, stroke, and chronic use of opioids; opioids have hypoventilatory effects. Diagnosis and treatment of hyperventilatory CSA may improve quality of life, and, when associated with heart failure or cerebrovascular disease, reduce morbidity and perhaps mortality.

Opioid-induced sleep disordered breathing presents a therapeutic predicament with the increasing incidence of prescription opioid use for noncancer chronic pain in the United States. Central sleep apnea with a Biot or cluster breathing pattern is characteristic of polysomnography studies; however, long-term clinical outcomes and the impact of therapy remain unknown. Novel ampakine-based therapies are being investigated. Randomized controlled trials with therapies that target the underlying pathophysiologic mechanisms of opioid-induced sleep disordered breathing are required.

# Preface

# The Development of Positive Airway Pressure Technology and Applications: Faster than Space Travel!

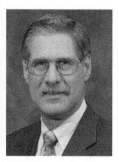  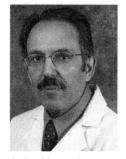

Lee K. Brown, MD         Shahrokh Javaheri, MD

*Editors*

The editorial focus of this issue of *Sleep Medicine Clinics* is to describe the rapid evolution of positive airway pressure (PAP) technology and the diverse applications of currently available devices. We are increasingly astounded by the capabilities that have been implemented since the vacuum cleaner blower and custom-fitted interface, first described by Sullivan in 1981, to the current availability of sophisticated devices having multiple operational modes. As an intellectual exercise, it is interesting to compare PAP development to that of spacecraft computational technology over a similar period. Contemporaneous with the origins of CPAP, the space shuttle program began with flight of *Columbia* on April 12, 1981 and ended in 2011. The space shuttles used, even after an upgrade, IBM AP-101S CPUs that could address only 256 kilobytes of memory and perform an underwhelming 1 million instructions per second (MIPS). The main computers equipping the American section of the International Space Station (ISS), still in active use, employ Intel 80386SX microprocessors. These chips were introduced in 1985, and when clocked at 33 MHz, could achieve about 11.4 MIPS and address up to 15 megabytes of memory; not bad for its time, but now sadly out of date. In comparison, beginning around the year 2000, Texas Instruments and other semiconductor manufacturers began marketing a series of CPUs (described as digital processing units in some literature) that could achieve performance far above that in the ISS. For instance, the Texas Instruments TMS320C2000 series that was marketed for use in CPAP generators starting around the year 2000 could run at clock speeds up to 300 MHz, perform up to 150 MIPS, had on-chip random access memory and flash (nonvolatile) memory of as much as 516 and 512 kilobytes, respectively (not both maxima in the same chip), along with on-chip functionalities that included analog-to-digital converters, pulse width modulation output for blower motor control, and an external memory bus to access additional memory. And that was 15 years ago and at a cost of no more than $20 each in quantity.

The exponential expansion of the functionality of CPUs available for commercial applications has been breathtaking to behold (see Moore's law). In parallel with this expansion, manufacturers of PAP flow generators have rapidly adapted to the strength of computing power now available in tiny form factors and at low prices in order to design flow generators with powerful capabilities that could not have been imagined by Sullivan in 1981. Yet, with great power comes great responsibility. The responsibility undertaken by physicians who prescribe these devices for the use of patients in their homes requires that they be mindful of the

Sleep Med Clin 12 (2017) xv–xvi
https://doi.org/10.1016/j.jsmc.2017.09.013
1556-407X/17/© 2017 Published by Elsevier Inc.

possibility that such complex devices may not behave as predicted when faced with the myriad patterns of sleep-disordered breathing that can occur in actual patients in the actual home setting. In this issue of *Sleep Medicine Clinics*, we have endeavored to comprehensively review PAP treatment for sleep-disordered breathing. We have included herein articles by leading experts in the field describing the technology employed by these devices, the choice of flow generator modality and patient interface, techniques for gaining patient acceptance of such treatment, and the nuances associated with the use of the current panoply of PAP generators in patients with a wide variety of conditions whose only similarity is that they exhibit some type (or many types) of sleep-disordered breathing. Our aim is thus to extend the Latin phrase *caveat emptor* ("let the buyer beware") to more specifically apply to the physician: *caveat medicus*.

Financial Disclosures: Dr Brown has participated in advisory panels for Philips Respironics and is an insurance claims reviewer for Considine and Associates, Inc. He co-edits the sleep and respiratory neurobiology section of *Current Opinion in Pulmonary Medicine*, wrote on CPAP treatment for obstructive sleep apnea in *UpToDate* and on obstructive sleep apnea in *Clinical Decision Support: Pulmonary Medicine and Sleep Disorders*. He is currently co-editing an issue of *Sleep Medicine Clinics* on positive airway pressure therapy. He serves on the Polysomnography Practice Advisory Committee of the New Mexico Medical Board and chairs the New Mexico Respiratory Care Advisory Board. Dr Javaheri has no relevant conflicts of interest.

Lee K. Brown, MD
Department of Internal Medicine
School of Medicine
University of New Mexico
Sleep Disorders Center
1101 Medical Arts Avenue Northeast, Building #2
Albuquerque, NM 87102, USA

Shahrokh Javaheri, MD
University of Cincinnati
Ohio University Medical School
Sleep Laboratory
Bethesda North Hospital
10475 Montgomery Road
Cincinnati, OH 45242, USA

*E-mail addresses:*
lkbrown@alum.mit.edu (L.K. Brown)
shahrokhjavaheri@icloud.com (S. Javaheri)

# Positive Airway Pressure Device Technology Past and Present
## What's in the "Black Box"?

Lee K. Brown, MD[a,b,*], Shahrokh Javaheri, MD[c,d,e]

## KEYWORDS

- Positive airway pressure • Obstructive sleep apnea • Central sleep apnea • Respiratory failure
- Noninvasive ventilation • Adaptive servo-ventilation • Volume assured pressure support

## KEY POINTS

- Fixed continuous positive airway pressure (CPAP) flow generators are now quiet, compact, and convenient.
- Autotitrating CPAP and bilevel PAP devices detect apneas and hypopneas and may distinguish between obstructive and central events. They treat obstructive and central sleep apnea while accommodating variations in the sleep-disordered breathing phenotype.
- Adaptive servo-ventilation can suppress the periodic breathing of Hunter–Cheyne–Stokes or central sleep apnea while simultaneously treating coexisting obstructive sleep-disordered breathing.
- Volume-assured pressure support technology can provide ventilatory support in the domiciliary setting for patients with a wide variety of breathing disorders.
- The complexity of the algorithms used can make it difficult to be sure how successfully targets are achieved.

## INTRODUCTION

The idea of applying positive pressure therapy in a noninvasive manner is not as recent as some might expect; in fact, the first reference to this treatment modality that is generally available appeared in *The Lancet* in 1936, reporting the use of positive pressure via facemask in the treatment of pulmonary

Financial Disclosures: L.K. Brown has participated in advisory panels for Philips Respironics, and is an insurance claims reviewer for Considine and Associates, Inc. He coedits the sleep and respiratory neurobiology section of *Current Opinion in Pulmonary Medicine*, wrote on continuous positive airway pressure treatment for obstructive sleep apnea in UpToDate, and on obstructive sleep apnea in *Clinical Decision Support: Pulmonary Medicine and Sleep Disorders*. He is currently coediting an issue of *Sleep Medicine Clinics* on positive airway pressure therapy. He serves on the Polysomnography Practice Advisory Committee of the New Mexico Medical Board and chairs the New Mexico Respiratory Care Advisory Board. S. Javaheri has no relevant conflict of interest.

[a] Division of Pulmonary, Critical Care, and Sleep Medicine, Department of Internal Medicine, University of New Mexico School of Medicine, University of New Mexico Sleep Disorders Center, 1101 Medical Arts Avenue NE, Building #2, Albuquerque, NM 87102, USA; [b] Department of Electrical and Computer Engineering, University of New Mexico School of Engineering, University of New Mexico Sleep Disorders Center, 1101 Medical Arts Avenue NE, Building #2, Albuquerque, NM 87102, USA; [c] Sleep Laboratory, Bethesda North Hospital, 10475 Montgomery Road, Cincinnati, OH 45242, USA; [d] TriHealth Sleep Center, Pulmonary and Sleep Division, Bethesda North Hospital, University of Cincinnati College of Medicine, 10500 Montgomery Road, Cincinnati, OH 45242, USA; [e] The Ohio State University College of Medicine, 473 West 12th Avenue, Columbus, OH 43210, USA
* Corresponding author. Department of Internal Medicine, School of Medicine, University of New Mexico, 1101 Medical Arts Avenue NE, Building #2, Albuquerque, NM 87102.
*E-mail address:* lkbrown@alum.mit.edu

Sleep Med Clin 12 (2017) 501–515
http://dx.doi.org/10.1016/j.jsmc.2017.07.001
1556-407X/17/© 2017 Elsevier Inc. All rights reserved.

edema.[1] Even more intriguing, Poulton makes reference to "artificial aerotherapeutics" having been described by Theodore Williams in Allbut and Rolleston's 1912 edition of *System of Medicine*, which I have unfortunately not been able to access. "Aerotherapeutics" is said by Poulton to include apparatus to "inflate or deflate the chest and lungs, and sometimes to carry out these processes alternately."[1] Over the ensuing years, numerous publications appeared describing the use of tight-fitting masks to achieve continuous positive airway pressure (CPAP), ventilatory support, and even ventilatory support with positive end-expiratory pressure (PEEP). Consequently, it is somewhat of a surprise that the idea of applying CPAP noninvasively to treat obstructive sleep apnea (OSA) did not emerge until the seminal report by Sullivan and colleagues[2] describing the application of CPAP via a custom nasal mask was published in 1981. Presumably, the confluence of the emerging recognition of obstructive sleep-disordered breathing (SDB), its high prevalence and effects on quality of life, along with the history of applying PAP via mask led the investigators to make the connection between these 2 threads of medical evolution. Whether this is an accurate portrayal of how the idea came to be, it is indisputable that CPAP and its various derivatives have proven to be a breakthrough in the treatment of OSA and, going forward, of other forms of SDB. Moreover, the availability of later generations of PAP apparatus made possible the routine use of noninvasive ventilation for patients with other forms of ventilatory failure, both acute and chronic as envisioned by Poulton.[1]

Following the description by Sullivan and colleagues,[2] the increasing use of CPAP for the treatment of OSA became a subject of major interest to entrepreneurs and led to the establishment of a growing cadre of manufacturers and the commercial availability of CPAP generators, masks, and accessories. This activity in turn drove the development of major improvements in PAP equipment, and the use of PAP for noninvasive ventilation added to the momentum of additional innovations. This article outlines the technology underlying the PAP equipment available commercially at the current time, focusing on the flow-generating element (generally described as the "blower"), the method for regulating the degree of positive pressure reaching the patient, the measurement of airflow received by the patient, and the use of the latter information to identify disordered breathing events, estimate minute ventilation versus mask leak, and use this information to establish a degree of closed circuit control of the patient's ventilation and breathing pattern. Much of the information herein

is proprietary and not released explicitly by the manufacturers. Much of the technology is described only in patent documents, and a degree of conjecture is involved in translating the information in the patents to the technology actually used in the various types of flow generators. In addition, the history of patents in PAP technology is convoluted, involving many claims and counterclaims, canceling of certain claims at a later date, and licensing agreements between manufacturers. For that reason, the authors make no claim that the patents referenced are the only documents describing a given technology nor were licensing arrangements required when similar technology was used by a manufacturer not identified as the assignee.

## BLOWERS AND CONTROL OF INTERFACE PRESSURE

It is perhaps of more than passing interest that the source of airflow used in the first report of CPAP treatment for OSA[2] used the blower from a vacuum cleaner, and this was the same source of airflow used in 1936 by Poulton[1] (in both cases, of course, using the outlet that normally served to exhaust the air that produced a vacuum). Both reports also used a means of controlling the volume of airflow, presumably by varying the voltage applied to drive the blower motors. Interestingly, Poulton used a more advanced method of providing a fixed value of positive pressure than did Sullivan and colleagues; Poulton placed what would in current terminology be identified as a PEEP valve, consisting of a spring-loaded bypass outlet fed separately from the tubing attached to the patient interface (mask). This bypass valve would open if the pressure exceeded a value that was set by the level of compression of the spring, thus maintaining a set degree of positive pressure. Sullivan and colleagues seem to have regulated pressure by varying the blower speed and the amount of resistance to airflow in series with the outlet flow to the tubing that led to the nasal mask, although shortly afterward, most systems used went back to controlling pressure with a PEEP valve.

The apparatus reported by Sullivan and colleagues clearly was not suitable for widespread deployment to treat the burgeoning number of patients being identified as suffering from OSA. According to a history of CPAP attributed to Sullivan and available on the ResMed website, the first CPAP apparatus available commercially used a "vortex blower" designed for jet or whirlpool baths. Such flow generators were heavy and noisy, attributes not particularly suited to use in a bedroom. These were alternating current

(AC) devices, and more difficult to control in terms of rotational speed (and thus airflow and ultimately pressure at the patient interface) than would a blower using a direct current (DC) motor. In addition, Sullivan's history does not provide information as to how a constant degree of positive pressure was maintained in the circuit, but it seems from his original US patent[3] that a second port for the exit of airflow was intended to be part of the nasal interface, and applied pressure would be controlled by varying the resistance of this exit port to airflow. (Note that in this patent reference and in all subsequent such references, there may exist conflicting patents of which we are not aware. Patent law is extremely complex and these references may not be generally accepted as controlling the use of the technology being described.) Clearly, such a method would not be capable of adapting to variations in mask pressure owing to changes in leak around the nasal interface, whether the patient was inhaling or exhaling, or the magnitude of the patient's minute ventilation. A better means was necessary to produce a more continuous degree of mask pressure, and one such method was essentially that introduced by Poulton mentioned earlier, that of incorporating a PEEP valve in the circuit to maintain mask pressure at a relatively fixed value.[1] Poulton attached the PEEP valve to the mask to prevent $CO_2$ rebreathing as did earlier CPAP devices. A more convenient location for the PEEP valve was made possible by the concept of incorporating a leak port in the mask (first introduced in a paper by Rapoport, in *Respiratory Management*, a journal no longer in publication[4]) and in a patent granted in 1991.[5] With a leak port built into the mask to prevent $CO_2$ rebreathing, the PEEP valve could then be placed anywhere in the airflow delivery circuit. One of us (L.K.B.) distinctly recalls a commercial CPAP device of that era that made provision for a PEEP valve fed by the patient circuit. The PEEP valves supplied were calibrated to provide specific level of PEEP in increments of 2.5 cm $H_2O$, and titration of CPAP, performed during nocturnal polysomnography (PSG), required swapping out the PEEP valves to provide progressively higher values of PEEP until the degree of positive pressure was achieved that alleviated the patient's OSA.

The next advance in blower technology occurred when the vortex fan was replaced by centrifugal designs powered by brushed 12-V DC motors. In essence, the brushes allowed for alternating the polarity of the DC current every 180° of rotation so that the motor could operate much like an AC device, with the added advantage that control of fan speed could be more easily accomplished by varying the DC voltage applied to the motor. Centrifugal designs were also quieter and lighter, although at first multistage devices were required to achieve the desired amount of airflow.[6] Further development resulted in single-stage designs that provided adequate airflow and were considerably smaller. Importantly, virtually every advance in PAP technology that followed depended on this ability to vary blower output by controlling the DC voltage applied to its motor.

Mask technology was originally quite primitive, requiring custom production of the mask by first producing a plaster cast of the patient's nose, from which a fiberglass mask conforming to that shape was produced. These masks were then glued to the patient's face each night to obtain a tight seal. However, mask technology was also rapidly advancing in parallel with blower technology, and an increasing variety of standard, manufactured interfaces began to be marketed that provided no standard degree of leak, either from a port designed to allow clearance of $CO_2$ and control mask pressure, nor from imperfect fitting of the mask to the patient's face. These included not only nasal masks, but also full face (oronasal) masks and even oral-only interfaces.[7–9] Given that circuit pressure could now be controlled by varying blower speed, the next obvious advance was to control blower speed by using a pressure sensor in the circuit that would produce a signal output that could control the blower speed via a closed feedback loop; this approach was patented in 1993 by Axe and colleagues[10] and assigned to the Board of Regents, The University of Texas System. This patent also contains the first mention, to our knowledge, of enlisting a microprocessor (an integrated circuit chip that is also known as a central processor unit or CPU in computer terminology) for use in the control circuitry of a CPAP generator. Microprocessors contain networks of transistors that accept digital data as input, process these data according to a program of instructions stored in its memory, and provide a digital output of the result. The patent by Axe and colleagues uses a microprocessor to receive pressure sensor data, calculate the necessary change in blower speed, and output control data to adjust the blower speed appropriately. In addition, direct control by a pressure sensor allowed for eliminating the known variation in system pressure that was prone to occur when the patient moved between significantly different altitudes, for example, back and forth between a sea-level city such as Los Angeles, California, to a mile-high city such as Albuquerque, New Mexico. Previously, CPAP generators had been provided with a switch that had 3 positions corresponding with low, medium, and high altitudes, although how the switch compensated for altitude changes is unclear.

It is likely that advances in semiconductor technology have eventually replaced the use of DC motors that incorporate brushes, as described, with circuits that supply a brushless motor with an AC current derived from the DC output of a switching power supply. These motors are also known as being electronically commutated, and yield multiple advantages: switching power supplies are considerably lighter and smaller than their analog counterparts; they are capable of operating seamlessly in countries that supply electricity at either 120 V AC/60 Hz or 240 V AC/50 Hz; and PAP generators can be designed to use the 12-V DC output of a switching power supply to power the fan as well as any associated electronics. That strategy allows for the use of the PAP device from a standard 12-V battery, such as when camping "off the grid." Moreover, suitable electronics can be used to control motor speed by altering the electronically commutated voltage waveform, amplitude, and frequency, yielding considerable additional flexibility. As proprietary information, it is not known how much of this capability is used in currently marketed PAP devices, although such use would be of no surprise.

## TAKING ADVANTAGE OF ADVANCED BLOWER TECHNOLOGY: RAMPING, BILEVEL POSITIVE AIRWAY PRESSURE, AND EXPIRATORY PRESSURE RELIEF

### Ramping

Unfortunately, initial compliance and long-term adherence to CPAP therapy can be problematic. One aspect of CPAP treatment that is not uncommonly a complaint of the new CPAP user is the difficulty tolerating the effort necessary to breathe out against the fixed pressure of the standard CPAP flow generator. Consequently, some patients report an inability to fall asleep if the prescribed pressure setting begins immediately upon activating the flow generator at the beginning of their sleep period. The DC-powered blower allowed for straightforward implementation of a "ramp" function: setting the CPAP generator to start at a lower, more tolerable pressure, and slowly ramping up to the prescribed pressure over a period of time chosen by the patient and/or prescribing practitioner, thus (theoretically) permitting the patient to fall asleep at a more comfortable degree of pressure and not reaching the higher, prescribed pressure until the patient was asleep.[11] There do not seem to be any studies, randomized controlled or otherwise, demonstrating that the ramp function improves

patient compliance or adherence to CPAP therapy,[12] although there is 1 report of so-called "ramp abuse" in which a patient continually restarts the ramp function during the course of the night, thereby preventing adequate treatment of the individual's OSA by not allowing sufficient sleep time with the device at the prescribed pressure.[13] Another issue with ramping that can mitigate against adequate treatment is ramp time. Some devices can be programmed for ramp times as long as 45 minutes, resulting in a significant period of time before pressure reaches a therapeutic level. As a consequence, the patient may fall asleep before adequate pressure is reached, prompting an awakening and preventing the onset of consolidated sleep. Some devices have algorithms that counter this deficiency by permitting the end-expiratory pressure to increase in response to obstructive events even while the ramp is in progress. Physicians using these devices need to be aware of the specific algorithm used by the prescribed device.

A technology that bears some resemblance to ramping was introduced in a report by Ayappa and colleagues[14] in 2009 and patented by Rapoport and Norman in 2006.[15] A neural network is configured to monitor the pattern of airflow so as to differentiate between regular breathing, SDB, REM sleep, and "troubled wakefulness." In theory, reducing the level of CPAP when "troubled wakefulness" is detected would result in a more comfortable experience and enhance compliance and adherence. One randomized controlled crossover trial is available comparing this strategy with autotitrating CPAP during one night's use of each modality in the sleep laboratory.[16] The study used the only currently marketed flow generator equipped with this technology (termed "SensAwake" and manufactured by Fisher & Paykel Healthcare Ltd, Auckland, NZ) but failed to demonstrate any differences in sleep architecture or patient satisfaction between the 2 modalities, although mean and 90th percentile pressures were lower in the wakefulness detection mode and apnea–hypopnea indices (AHI) were similar. Clearly, more extended randomized controlled trials will be necessary to determine whether this technology improves compliance and adherence.

### Bilevel Positive Airway Pressure

The genesis of expiratory pressure relief (EPR) technology and bilevel PAP flow generators are inextricably bound together, and depend on the theory that airway collapse is primarily an inspiratory event and that a lower (or no) degree of expiratory pressure was necessary as long as inspiratory PAP (IPAP) could stent the airway open at the beginning of inhalation. It seems that bilevel PAP was introduced commercially before EPR, and therefore is discussed first. Both technologies depend on the ability to detect breath phase to modulate the degree of pressure introduced to the patient interface, depending on whether the phase is inspiratory versus expiratory. This was a relatively simple matter for mechanical ventilation via an endotracheal tube or other direct connection to the airway, because the inspiratory and expiratory paths for flow are separate and little in the way of air leak occurs if the direct airway connection is secure. Breath phase can then be determined from pressure or flow in each limb of the ventilatory circuit, allowing for the application of PEEP and many other specialized forms of ventilation. The situation with noninvasive application of PAP is more complicated, in that there are no separate inspiratory and expiratory limbs and there is a deliberate amount of leak (intentional leak) from the patient interface that allows for the clearance of exhaled $CO_2$. The breakthrough technology is documented in 2 patents by Sanders and Zdrojkowski that were granted in 1989[17] and 1992[18] and the clinical use of bilevel PAP in OSA is described in the seminal paper by Sanders and Kern in 1990.[19] The method consists of inserting a flow sensor in the output circuit of the blower that produces a voltage proportional to the flow. Assuming no radical change in interface leakage, the average signal from that transducer equals the leakage flow, because inspiration will increase system flow to the same extent that expiration will decrease system flow. This average flow rate is then electronically compared with instantaneous flow. An increase in instantaneous flow compared with average flow then signals the onset of inspiration, whereas a decrease in instantaneous flow compared with average flow signals the onset of expiration; the signal from the electronic comparator changes depending on whether inspiration or expiration is detected and governs the alternation between IPAP and expiratory PAP (EPAP). It is then possible for this signal to initiate a blower speed during inspiration to provide IPAP and a lower blower speed during expiration to provide EPAP. It should be mentioned that, over the years, more sophisticated methods of filtering, averaging, and otherwise processing these signals emerged that improved the accuracy of breath phase determination. Also, this description is relevant only for bilevel PAP in the spontaneous (triggered) mode. Bilevel PAP devices set to a spontaneous/timed mode use timing circuitry that initiates a transition to IPAP if a set period of time passes without detection of an inspiration,

and bilevel PAP in timed mode simply does away with the detection of respiratory phase and the switch between EPAP and IPAP is only governed by a timer set to produce a certain respiratory rate. Finally, when a microprocessor is involved in the overall control of the system, a repertoire of additional features can be implemented: triggering threshold, IPAP or EPAP that deviates from constant levels but varies over time (eg, increase time for IPAP), and variations in the inspiratory/expiratory ratio, to name but a few. It also must be mentioned that methods have been developed, to be described elsewhere in this paper, to estimate actual instantaneous patient airflow. The strategy developed by Sanders and Zdrojkowski that led to the development of bilevel PAP continues to be used in modern flow generators, although digital filtering has replaced the analog methods originally used. The digital approach also makes possible the design of flow generators that have the ability to be set to a variety of modes, starting with fixed CPAP but extending to adaptive servo-ventilation (ASV) and average volume assured pressure support (PS).

Sanders and Kern postulated that the use of bilevel PAP could reduce the overall degree of pressure necessary to prevent both obstructive apneas and hypopneas, and therefore would be more comfortable for the patient; that, in turn, could improve patient adherence to therapy. Whether bilevel PAP does indeed improve adherence in OSA patients is beyond the scope of this paper, although many of us in clinical practice can attest to the fact that some patients seem to tolerate bilevel PAP better than CPAP. Perhaps the most significant impact of bilevel PAP, however, is not related to the treatment of patients with OSA but with the use of the technology for ventilatory support. Moreover, the indications for the use of bilevel PAP for ventilatory support have broadened considerably over the last few decades. Noninvasive positive pressure ventilation using a variety of oral or nasal contrivances had been in routine use by some practitioners for many years. This was accomplished using standard volume or pressure ventilators, and was applied to patients with chronic ventilatory failure that was usually due to neuromuscular or neurologic disease. It seems that the earliest report of the use of the then commercially available bilevel PAP for ventilatory support was that of Robertson and Roloff in 1994, who treated 2 patients with chronic ventilatory failure from muscular dystrophy.[20] No doubt the availability of a variety of commercially available interfaces, initially developed for CPAP treatment, facilitated this new application of bilevel PAP. The rest, as they say, is history, because bilevel PAP is now used not just to treat chronic ventilatory failure of many etiologies, but for many forms of acute respiratory decompensation as well.

## Expiratory Pressure Relief

The same technology that allowed for the determination of ventilatory phase, as well as the flexibility in pressure control made possible by the incorporation of microprocessors, undoubtedly led to the concept of adding EPR capability to CPAP flow generators. EPR is thus a generic term that can accurately be applied to bilevel PAP, C-flex (as marketed by Philips Respironics, Inc., Murrysville, PA), and the altered expiratory pressure waveform incorporated by ResMed and other vendors in their PAP generators. The use of bilevel PAP for EPR has already been discussed; this section focuses on C-flex and other modalities of EPR used by the major manufacturers. The earliest patent applicable to this concept seems to have been filed in 1996 by Estes and Fiore, in which they describe a method to modulate applied pressure based on the patient's degree of airflow.[21] Nilius and colleagues[22] published the first report of the actual use of what they referred to as pressure-relief CPAP in 2006 and used a Philips Respironics flow generator with the option referred to as C-flex. With C-flex, the pressure was decreased in expiration only during the period of flow, as opposed to bilevel PAP, in which the lower level of EPAP is maintained during all of expiration. The magnitude of the pressure decrease in response to airflow is adjustable to a certain degree by the operator selecting values of 1, 2, or 3 for the C-flex setting, although the exact effect of the different settings is not explained other than that the higher the number, the greater the magnitude of the C-flex pressure change. The original C-flex devices were marketed as a means to increase patient comfort, without providing a detailed explanation of the physiologic principle. Eventually, it became apparent that the drop in expiratory pressure was being titrated to flow because this kept the pressure at the collapsible segment of the airway constant and at the necessary pressure to offset the "tissue pressure" (which follows from the Starling model) without ever going above it; an additional component of expiratory pressure was provided by upstream resistance to expiratory airflow, primarily from nasal resistance. The presumption was that doing so would enhance compliance and adherence to CPAP treatment. However, detailed evaluation of pressures at the mask and the supraglottic region by Masdeu and colleagues[23] suggest that C-flex does not actually

mitigate supraglottic pressure and therefore may not achieve its intended purpose. Indeed, the most recent (2009) Cochrane metaanalysis of the effects of pressure relief technologies on CPAP adherence did not find any significant difference when any of these modalities were used compared with fixed CPAP.[24]

Most likely based on patents filed in 2005 and 2010 by Bassin and issued in the United States in 2011 and 2014,[25,26] and assigned to ResMed Limited (New South Wales, Australia), ResMed introduced its own version of EPR. Because Philips Respironics held the patent for EPR governed by expiratory airflow, ResMed took the approach of lowering EPAP at the beginning of expiration to enhance patient comfort, and then following a predetermined pattern until the end of expiration. Because it is not governed by airflow, ResMed EPR resembles bilevel PAP to a great degree. According to the patents, the pressure versus time function is determined by an estimate of the expiratory duration. The degree of EPR at the beginning of expiration, according to the patents, is a function of the pressure required during inspiration; that is, the higher the CPAP pressure required to fully treat the patient's OSA, the greater the degree of initial EPR. The patents suggest that a typical value of EPR would be 3 cm $H_2O$, but commercial devices also incorporate an adjustment that also affects the amount of EPR. This adjustment is typically delineated by numerical values between 1 and 3, with 3 yielding the highest amount of EPR. However, the actual value of EPR corresponding with these numerical settings in not available and the setting is determined empirically, generally by querying the patient about their degree of comfort with breathing out against pressure and choosing an EPR setting accordingly. In our experience, this commonly results in the technologist routinely setting the EPR to "3," which has also been our experience with C-flex.

It deserves repeating that the most recent (2009) Cochrane metaanalysis of the effects of pressure relief technologies on CPAP adherence did not find any significant difference when either EPR or bilevel PAP was used compared with fixed CPAP.[21]

## AUTOTITRATING FLOW GENERATORS
### Autotitrating Continuous Positive Airway Pressure

In the early 1990s, a quest began to develop CPAP flow generators that could detect apneas, hypopneas, and (in some cases) snoring, and automatically adjust the degree of pressure delivered to the patient. As the field of sleep medicine advanced and clinicians became aware of the significance of CSA, it became apparent that it would be necessary for these devices to also distinguish between central (open airway) respiratory events and obstructive apneas and hypopneas, because increasing CPAP levels in response to central events often proves to be counterproductive. Previous to this development, CPAP was administered at a fixed pressure almost always determined during PSG, and the goal was to determine a pressure that was effective in all sleep positions and stages, particularly during supine REM sleep, when OSA is typically more severe. It was widely assumed, although evidence is scant, that the higher the pressure, the greater was the likelihood that the patient would be intolerant of CPAP, and hence the development of the bilevel PAP and EPR technologies as detailed. It was felt that if an autotitrating CPAP device was available, pressures would vary according to the needs of the patient at various points in time during the night, that is, lower pressure during nonsupine sleep and/or lower pressure during non-REM sleep. Consequently, the patient would receive, on average, lower pressures during the course of the night and would experience fewer of the side effects known to be related to higher pressures. Autotitrating CPAP would also allow the treatment pressure to vary as needed, not just during the course of a single night, but also compensate for night-to-night, week-to-week, and even longer term variations in pressure requirements. Such variations were known to occur in the early stages of CPAP treatment owing to a reduction in upper airway edema, as well as on a longer term basis with weight gain or loss, nasal congestion from allergic rhinitis or upper respiratory infections, and ingestion of alcohol or other drugs near to sleep (eg, opioids).[27] Although not known at the time, specific populations (patients with heart failure, chronic kidney disease, or end-stage renal disease) could also require increasingly higher levels of CPAP during course of the night owing to fluid shifts, particularly from the lower extremities, resulting in upper airway edema. Other justifications included obviating the need for titration during a PSG, especially in locations where sleep laboratory services are not readily available or when high demand leads to long delays in scheduling a laboratory titration. Finally, the increasing use of split-night protocols during PSG, wherein a diagnostic phase is followed by CPAP titration during a single night of testing, was perceived as being more likely to result in a less-than-satisfactory titration owing to time constraints.

Examination of the patents applicable to autotitrating technology illustrates the variety of strategies that were developed to detect apneas, hypopneas, and snoring; and much later on (when the importance of distinguishing open airway events from obstructive events was recognized), techniques to distinguish between the 2 mechanisms. The earliest autotitrating devices undoubtedly depended on the technology described for bilevel PAP to detect apneas: comparing average airflow delivered to the patient with the changes in flow engendered by tidal breathing. When no tidal breathing is detected for 10 seconds or longer, an apnea is identified. This approach is described in a patent assigned to ResMed Limited, (North Ryde, Australia) that was filed in 1998 and granted in 2002.[28] An earlier patent, assigned to ResMed's predecessor corporation, ResCare Limited (also in North Ryde, Australia) describes an apnea detection method that depends on pressure measurements at the patient interface that are processed to extract a signal indicating snoring and a signal indicating airflow.[29] To our knowledge, that technique never resulted in a commercially marketed product. Its relevance, however, may be that it represents one of the earliest patents of technology for autotitration of CPAP.

The next obstacle involved the detection of hypopneas—because, as the field advanced, the importance of these respiratory events became apparent (even though the 2 types of SDB continue to be called "obstructive sleep apnea" and "central sleep apnea"). A patent granted to Axe and colleagues[30] in 1995 seems to be the first report of a method for detecting hypopneas as well as apneas from reductions, rather than absences, of the flow signal, respectively. Another method, involving detection of inspiratory flow limitation, was also proposed early on but not adopted until much later in the development of autotitrating technology. The adoption of this latter technology was prompted by the need to distinguish between open airway events that could be central apneas or hypopneas, and those associated with some degree of upper airway obstruction, either partial (obstructive hypopneas) or total (obstructive apneas). The subject of inspiratory flow limitation is discussed in detail elsewhere in this article.

A variety of techniques have been developed to determine whether the mechanism responsible for any given event is obstructive or central, because an increase in CPAP in response to a central apnea or hypopnea is usually counterproductive.

Three methods, usually in some combination, are commonly used for this determination: detection of snoring, identification of a cardiac artifact superimposed on the flow signal, and measurement of upper airway resistance using forced oscillation.

Detection and analysis of snoring was, and continues to be, used in autotitrating devices. Earlier autotitrating CPAP flow generators depended heavily on this methodology, which involves bandpass filtering of the flow in the patient circuit (the same flow that is measured within the device in the techniques detailed) to detect energy in a frequency spectrum associated with snoring.[31] Initially, a snore was considered as an indicator of an impending apnea, and this information was used to determine whether an increase in CPAP was indicated. In isolation, this methodology proved to be insufficient for accurate titration of CPAP. However, snoring detection and analysis remains an integral part of the algorithms used in the autotitrating flow generators marketed by some manufacturers. Usually, snoring detection is combined with other methods to identify obstructive hypopneas, and spectral analysis of the flow signal can be used to determine the degree of upper airway narrowing associated with a hypopnea.[32] One drawback of using snoring only in this application is the finding that snoring tends to decrease in intensity during REM sleep owing to the reduction in inspiratory effort that is common in this sleep stage.[33]

Reference to the generation of small amounts of airflow in the airways coincident with cardiac filling and contraction date back to at least 1942, as described by Luisada,[34] and such artifacts were observed repeatedly during various types of pulmonary physiologic testing over the years, such as associated with the single-breath nitrogen washout maneuver. The observation of cardiac artifact in the flow signal during PSG and whether it was indicative of central apneas engendered a certain degree of controversy during the latter part of the 1990s,[35] which was somewhat put to rest by Ayappa and colleagues[36] in a study demonstrating a high degree of correlation between the presence of this finding and apneas of central mechanism. Even before this definitive study the concept had been patented for use in autotitrating CPAP,[37] and several additional patents quickly followed.[38,39] Interestingly, the patent documents often indicate that detection of the cardiac flow artifact was to be combined with a second method of determining airway patency, namely, the forced oscillation technique. Despite the findings of Ayappa and colleagues,[36] the findings of Morrell and colleagues[35] clearly brought

into question whether the detection of cardiac artifact in the flow signal was sufficient evidence of an open airway apnea. Forced oscillation methodology also has a long history, dating back to a publication by DuBois and associates in 1956.[40] In practice, a pressure is generated that alternates at a frequency significantly higher than the normal respiratory rate and is impressed upon normal ventilation. The resulting flow signal is extracted and a variety of calculations are then possible that use the pressure and flow signals to determine several measurements of the respiratory system that are analogous to parameters commonly used in electrical circuit analysis, namely, impedance, which is a value that combines resistance and reactance. Resistance applies to the flow induced by an imposed pressure that is constant; reactance is a measurement that is determined by the compliance and inertance of the respiratory system. Impedance may be expressed as the magnitude of flow created by the alternating pressure and the phase difference between the pressure and flow waveforms; alternatively, it may be expressed as a real number (the resistance) plus or minus an imaginary number (the reactance, consisting of a real number multiplied by $j$, which is the square root of $-1$). Because the reactance component can generally be ignored for the purpose of determining whether the airway is open or closed in this application, autotitrating devices typically use only the absolute value of flow provoked by the impressed alternating pressure as a measure of airway patency.[31,32]

In addition to obstructive hypopnea detection using analysis of a snoring signal, hypopneas are also identified by reductions in flow that do not achieve the cutoff level associated with recognition of an apnea. As mentioned, these flow signals are subject to a variety of averaging, filtering, and other processing to more accurately detect a sufficient degree of airflow reduction that merits identification of a hypopnea. Moreover, information from the forced oscillation signal can also be used to measure degrees of upper airway impedance that indicate partial obstruction. Perhaps more frequently, however, the shape of the inspiratory flow curve is used to identify partial airway obstruction and thus an obstructive hypopnea. Flattening of the inspiratory limb of the maximal inspiratory/expiratory flow–volume loop as recorded during spirometry in the pulmonary function laboratory has long been associated with variable upper airway flow limitation.[41] It was later recognized that the same phenomenon could be observed during tidal breathing in infants with variable upper airway obstruction,[42] and Condos and colleagues[43] followed by Sériès and

Marc[44] found that tidal breathing during sleep demonstrated flattening of the inspiratory limb in patients with OSA. A few years earlier, patents by Rapoport and Norman described the use of inspiratory limb flattening to identify upper airway narrowing during CPAP treatment and use that finding to control the titration of CPAP.[45,46] This method, or more complicated techniques analyzing the shape of the inspiratory limb of tidal breathing during sleep,[47] have become the mainstay of obstructive hypopnea identification to titrate CPAP automatically. Moreover, the various methodologies are almost always combined in a "layered" or multifaceted algorithm to determine whether, in what direction, and to what degree, a CPAP change is warranted. Examination of the flow charts in one of the previously referenced patents should be sufficient to inform the reader as to the potential complexity of the algorithms being used to autotitrate CPAP.[32]

### Autotitrating Bilevel Positive Airway Pressure

It was inevitable that manufacturers of autotitrating CPAP flow generators would eventually apply the same technology to bilevel PAP. Surprisingly, the available devices operate only in spontaneous mode, and it is necessary to prescribe ASV if a timed mode is necessary. Some devices allow only a fixed EPAP that could presumably be determined during a PSG, either by identifying the CPAP level that was sufficient to suppress obstructive apneas but not hypopneas, or by actually titrating the EPAP setting of an autotitrating bilevel PAP during another PSG. All marketed devices titrate IPAP within a bound set by specifying a maximum amount of PS, although not every flow generator allows the specification of a minimum amount of PS. A device that will autotitrate EPAP is also available, presumably by incorporating the apnea detection technology from that manufacturer's autotitrating CPAP devices.

These autotitrating bilevel PAP devices incorporate a high degree of complexity (and therefore introduce the possibility of unpredictable results) of the algorithms to titrate EPAP in the presence of a nonconstant baseline pressure that defines bilevel. When one wishes to go beyond eliminating apnea and hypopnea, the calculations of inspiratory flow shape that underlie the best forms of autotitration of CPAP (and EPAP in bilevel PAP) are totally dependent on a fixed (or calculable) driving pressure. The calculations during changing driving pressure, along with a host of assumptions, allow one in principle to calculate the portion of inspiration that is machine driven, and that which

is patient driven. These assumptions and calculations are very complex and frequently fail when the leak of the mask or through the mouth changes, and when the mask balloons out under IPAP. Most autotitration of bilevel EPAP is (at least for some patients) questionable, and this is most problematic when it comes to the autotitration of EPAP for the treatment of residual subtle obstruction. The choice of IPAP is also difficult to titrate when there is hypoventilation because there is no clear signal for "adequate" ventilation. In the case of ASV, a target amount of ventilation or flow is incorporated, making ASV a much more successful modality, because the goal is often just stabilizing ventilation with minimal need for EPAP.

### ADAPTIVE SERVO-VENTILATION

The development of new medical technology is inevitably the result of the need to treat a particular disorder for which available modalities are not effective. In the case of ASV, the need was that patients with congestive heart failure or who have suffered a cerebrovascular accident often exhibit a pattern of breathing first described by John Hunter and most accurately referred to as Hunter–Cheyne–Stokes breathing (HCSB). This breathing pattern consists of repetitive cycles of crescendo–decrescendo changes in tidal breathing with central apneas or hypopneas interposed between the intervals of ventilation. These same patients may, instead, exhibit central sleep apnea without the HCSB pattern, and central sleep apnea may also be idiopathic in nature. Both breathing patterns are the result of ventilatory control instability, manifesting as a cycling of the respiratory drive, the etiology of which is beyond the scope of this article, but has been reviewed elsewhere.[48] The theory behind ASV holds that it acts to counterbalance this ventilatory instability by varying the degree of PS out of phase with the patient's own ventilatory drive, thus acting to dampen the factors leading to periodic breathing. ASV also stabilizes the upper airway to prevent obstructive apneas by applying a fixed or variable EPAP, just as in conventional bilevel PAP.[49] These devices also apply mandatory breaths in a timed backup mode as necessary, and these multiple strategies for suppressing HCSB, central sleep apnea, and OSA make ASV technology potentially effective in the treatment of hybrid forms of SDB that are a combination of both central and obstructive events. In addition, ASV can be viewed as another pressure relief technology that could be useful in treating patients with OSA who are intolerant of CPAP with or without EPR and bilevel PAP.

It is impossible to describe the technology used in ASV without separately describing the flow generators marketed by the major suppliers of these devices in the United States, namely, ResMed and Philips Respironics. As described in the relevant patents, ResMed devices determine instantaneous respiratory airflow by first estimating instantaneous mask leak, and then subtracting this from total mask airflow.[50] Instantaneous mask leak is computed by measuring instantaneous mask airflow and pressure in the patient circuit within the device, and applying low-pass filtering to eliminate high-frequency noise. Instantaneous mask airflow is divided by the square root of instantaneous mask pressure to obtain a measure of conductance, and mask leak is then derived from this conductance multiplied by the square root of the instantaneous mask pressure. Instantaneous respiratory airflow can then be determined by subtracting mask leak from total flow. The patient's recent average ventilation is obtained by continuously computing the absolute value of a 100-second period of low-pass filtered instantaneous respiratory airflow. A low-pass filter with such a long time constant is essentially computing the integral of the instantaneous respiratory airflow and the result is a value proportional to average ventilation. The patent document specifies that the length of the time constant is chosen to exceed the typical lung–chemoreceptor delay time as well as the typical cycle time for HCSB.[50] This choice of time constant is thought to better suppress periodic breathing without requiring an excessive delay before convergence on a steady-state degree of ventilation. Shorter time constants could result in less stability and longer time constants could delay arriving at an equilibrium condition.

A percentage of this recent average ventilation is then used as the target input in a regulatory control loop programmed into the microprocessor and configured as a negative feedback controller. The patent document specifies that 90% to 95% of the recent average ventilation is used, although published investigations and reviews that describe the ResMed device seem to consistently mention 90%,[51–53] as did the manufacturer's informational material, which seem to no longer be available on the Internet. According to the patent, using an excessive percentage of recent average ventilation results in positive feedback and drift in the steady-state level of ventilation, and an insufficient percentage may not fully suppress HCSB. The absolute value of the instantaneous respiratory airflow is also sampled by the microprocessor acting as an integral clipped controller, meaning its output is both integrated over a period of time

and bounded so as not to fall below a minimum value and not to exceed a maximum value. The output is an error term consisting of the absolute value of instantaneous respiratory airflow minus the target value multiplied by a constant and integrated over several breaths so as to ensure that variations in PS from the device are opposite in phase to the patient's own variations in ventilatory drive; that is, maximum PS occurs when the patient's ventilatory drive is at a minimum and minimum PS occurs when the patient's own ventilatory drive has peaked. The patent states a typical value for the constant used by the integral controller of $-0.3$ cm $H_2O$ per L/min per second.[50] Finally, the microprocessor uses the instantaneous respiratory airflow signal to judge respiratory phase and thus determine transitions between EPAP and IPAP (ie, when to supply PS). The patent offers 2 methods to identify phase: one is simply based on the sign of instantaneous respiratory airflow, and the other uses the sign of the instantaneous respiratory airflow and its rate of change to determine "fuzzy" categories of respiratory phase. In addition, the 5-second low-pass filtered absolute value of instantaneous respiratory airflow is used to determine whether the patient is exhibiting a regular respiratory rate or requires a timed backup rate. The manufacturer's literature, also seeming to be no longer available, stated that the device assesses the "instantaneous direction, magnitude, and rate of change of the patient's airflow," implying that the second, more complicated method is implemented in the marketed device. The first generation of ResMed ASV devices, as used in the SERVE-HF trial,[54] incorporated fixed EPAP but currently available flow generators incorporate the ability to titrate EPAP. This regulation is accomplished in a manner similar to that used in their autotitrating CPAP devices.

As with the ResMed device, The Philips Respironics ASV flow generators use an estimate of instantaneous patient air flow as the basis for the control algorithm. The patent does not describe the specific manner in which this is done,[55] although prior patents incorporated by reference specify 2 possible techniques.[56] The more simple method involves computing instantaneous air flow averaged over multiple breaths that is taken to represent average leak, because inspiratory and expiratory tidal volumes will sum to zero. Instantaneous air flow, when subtracted from this average flow, then represents an estimate of instantaneous patient air flow. The other method for estimating instantaneous patient air flow is similar to that used in the ResMed flow generator. Rather than computing leak pathway conductance on an instantaneous basis, Philips Respironics apparently computes this value averaged over an entire breath and then computes the instantaneous mask leak air flow by multiplying this average conductance by the square root of the instantaneous circuit pressure. Subtracting this value from instantaneous system air flow then results in an estimate of instantaneous patient air flow. It may be that the former method is used in controlling transitions between EPAP and IPAP as well as computing the patient's respiratory rate, and the latter technique is used in the pressure control algorithm.

Assuming that all aspects of the process described in the patent are actually implemented in the marketed device, the procedure for controlling IPAP for any given breath is quite complex.[55] The objective is to achieve a target peak flow by comparing this value with the measured peak flow for each breath. The value of IPAP for the next breath is then adjusted so as to reach that target, within the constraints of maximum and minimum IPAP as set by the provider. There are 3 parameters involved: an HCSB shape index, HCSB severity index, and a PS index. The PS index is perhaps easiest to understand, in that it is simply the percentage of breaths during the previous 2 to 3 minutes (or, alternatively, the previous 2 HCSB cycles) that required a value of PS above a threshold level (typically 2 cm $H_2O$, as stated in the patent). Both HCSB indices are derived from an array of peak flows collected over the previous 2 to 5 minutes. The array of peak flows are filtered to ensure that they vary above and below a zero flow point; 3 zero crossings are detected and used to identify 2 putative sequences of HCSB. The peak flows are then compared with a standard template of peak flows (the patent describes using a triangle function, but presumably other functions could be used) that models an extreme degree of HCSB, and a coherence value is computed that ranges between 0% and 100%; this is considered to be a measure of how closely the actual array of peak flows conforms to the template's model of severe HCSB. Finally, the HCSB severity index is computed as the ratio of the last minimum peak flow over the last maximum peak flow, or an average of these ratios over a set interval is converted to a percentage that ranges between 0% and 100%. A severity index of 50% or greater is considered "normal," meaning that peak flow during normal breathing may vary to that degree; values of less than 50% indicate the presence of HCSB, with a value of zero representing the occurrence of a central apnea. The actual computation that determines changes in IPAP for each breath incorporates 3 factors: a target peak flow, an

adjustment using the 3 parameters as described, and the difference between the previous breath's peak flow and the target peak flow multiplied by a constant ("gain") that is nominally 9 cm $H_2O$/L per second. In addition, the amount that IPAP changes with each breath is proportional to this difference value, so that large discrepancies between actual and target peak flow result in greater changes in IPAP then would result from small differences in this metric.

Two backup rate mechanisms are available, or the device can be set to spontaneous mode only. One mechanism allows for a provider-chosen backup respiratory rate, and the other calculates the patient's customary respiratory rate and adds a machine breath when excessive time passes without a spontaneous breath. Philips Respironics also uses several proprietary methods to determine cycling between EPAP and IPAP. Transitions from EPAP to IPAP occur when either an accumulated inspired volume of 6 mL is detected, or when expiratory air flow crosses a transformed flow waveform called the "shape signal." The latter is the patient's actual flow decreased by a constant 15 L/min and delayed by a constant 300 msec. This method is said to allow trigger sensitivity to adjust to different values of leak and spontaneous breathing patterns. Transitions from IPAP to EPAP are also governed in 2 ways: during inspiration, when instantaneous patient air flow falls below a value proportional to instantaneous tidal volume, or when time in IPAP exceeds 3.0 seconds.

## VOLUME-ASSURED PRESSURE SUPPORT

The earliest report of the noninvasive use of volume-assured PS (VAPS) ventilation was its application for the treatment of OSA, rather than as a ventilatory support mode.[57] Unfortunately, the manufacturer sponsoring this research did not choose to further develop the technology, perhaps owing to the increasing success of more conventional forms of PAP for treatment of OSA and not realizing the potential for the use of noninvasive VAPS for outpatient ventilatory support. The justification for noninvasive VAPS in the outpatient setting is often given as the ability for the device to maintain a given level of ventilatory support without underventilating or overventilating the patient. Absent the ability to measure $Paco_2$ or a surrogate (end-tidal $Pco_2$, which is not reliable in patients with significant airways disease, or transcutaneous $Pco_2$, which is virtually impossible to deploy in the outpatient setting) to control the level of ventilatory support, the main advantage of noninvasive VAPS is the ability to compensate for possible changes in respiratory mechanics. Bilevel PAP does not have this capability, but this does not seem to have hindered its widespread deployment in patients with chronic ventilatory failure, including those prone to variations in respiratory mechanics such as patients with chronic obstructive pulmonary disease.

That being said, the VAPS technology is available and is increasingly being prescribed, and consequently the underlying technology should be understood. Once again, a review of the applicable patents is instructive. The most relevant patents in the case of the Philips Respironics average VAPS product incorporates by reference the technology for determining instantaneous patient airflow previously described with respect to ASV.[58,59] Therefore, the methodology for measuring leakage airflow and instantaneous patient airflow is presumably the same as in their ASV devices. The patents specify that a target tidal volume is set by the prescribing practitioner, and PS is adjusted on a breath-by-breath basis to achieve this target. The algorithm does this by comparing the tidal volume averaged over 2 to 6 breath cycles and then increases or decreases PS for the subsequent breath to achieve the target tidal volume. There have been a variety of methods used in the published literature to determine the target tidal volume, including based on ideal body weight (as recommended by the manufacturer and calculated from height), measurement of $Paco_2$ either by arterial blood gas determination or transcutaneous $Pco_2$ (awake or asleep), or by determining a level which is "comfortable" for the patient and then setting the goal 110% higher.[60–65] Per the manufacturer, the respiratory rate is set to between 2 and 3 breaths/min below the patient's resting rate and together with the set tidal volume, specify a target minute ventilation. A version of the Philips Respironics average VAPS (AVAPS-AE) is also available that piggybacks the ability to simultaneously titrate EPAP using the technology as described.

The ResMed version of VAPS is marketed as iVAPS, ("i" is stated by the manufacturer as indicating "intelligent") and again seems to use much the same technology as their ASV device to determine instantaneous patient airflow, leak, and respiratory phase (in this case, respiratory phase seems to be determined using the "fuzzy" logic technique).[66] The target alveolar ventilation (as described elsewhere in this article), is achieved by varying the degree of PS for each breath to produce a tidal volume that, when multiplied by the respiratory rate, reaches the ventilatory target. The respiratory rate is determined by measuring the patients native respiratory rate, and a backup

rate is computed as two-thirds of the native respiratory rate so that it only comes into play when the patient fails to trigger a ventilator breath after a set period of time.[67] The target for the ResMed device is specified as alveolar ventilation rather than tidal volume, and according to ResMed's website, the value is calculated by subtracting an estimate of dead space ventilation from a minute ventilation target, which can either be estimated by specifying the patient's height, or by using "disease-specific preset values (for obstructive, restrictive, normal lung mechanics and obesity hypoventilation) based on commonly used clinical values."[68] In addition, the iVAPS device incorporates a "learning" mode, which is described as a specified period of (presumably awake) time during which the device measures the patient's native respiratory rate and tidal volume, and computes a target minute ventilation from these data.[69,70] Presumably, many of these parameters can be set manually, as is described in a report by Oscroft and colleagues[71] wherein iVAPS was used in the domiciliary treatment of chronic obstructive pulmonary disease. As is the case with the Philips Respironics device, the target minute ventilation can also be determined by measuring $Paco_2$ either by arterial blood gas determination or transcutaneous $Pco_2$ (awake or asleep), or by assessment of patient comfort at a particular setting. Finally, currently available information indicates that EPAP is manually set and autotitration of this parameter is not (yet) incorporated in ResMed's VAPS device.

## SUMMARY

The astute reader will note that we have not attempted to describe the algorithms followed by the autotitrating devices to achieve their goals. The algorithms can be extremely complex, and in any case are subject to change by the manufacturer as products are updated or new models are introduced. We have also not attempted, particularly with respect to autotitrating CPAP, to specify the measurements that any particular model uses in its algorithm. There is a recent publication that does incorporate such information for some of the current models of autotitrating devices, and the reader may possibly rely on this source for some inkling of this information.[72]

All of the autotitrating devices described have the ability to measure and store a variety of adherence data as well as estimates of leak and AHI, including in some cases distinguishing between apneas and hypopneas and central versus obstructive mechanism. These data are derived from the same technology that is controlling the treatment parameters, and therefore there is a degree of circularity in play: the device is essentially determining its own effectiveness. We have already commented on the inability of some autotitrating devices to properly respond to SDB patterns created by respiratory simulators in an earlier editorial.[73] More recently, the American Thoracic Society reviewed the literature concerning accuracy of the residual AHI reported by autotitrating flow generators. This Official Statement urged caution with respect to placing undue faith on the residual AHIs derived from such downloads.[74] It would be wise to remember that if an autotitrating device is reporting satisfactory effectiveness but the patient is still symptomatic, it may be desirable to independently verify that the device is effectively controlling the patient's SDB by PSG monitoring in the laboratory.

## ACKNOWLEDGMENTS

The authors thank Dr David Rapoport for contributing his insights into the history of positive airway pressure technology. As an individual responsible for many of the major advances in this technology, his intimate knowledge of the subject was invaluable.

## REFERENCES

1. Poulton EP. Left sided heart failure with pulmonary edema; its treatment with the pulmonary plus pressure machine. Lancet 1936;228:981–3.
2. Sullivan CE, Issa FG, Berthon-Jones M, et al. Reversal of obstructive sleep apnoea by continuous positive airway pressure applied through the nares. Lancet 1981;1(8225):862–5.
3. Sullivan CE, inventor; Somed Pty Ltd, assignee. Device for treating snoring sickness. US patent 4,944,310. July 31, 1990.
4. Rapoport DM. Techniques for administering nasal CPAP. Respir Manage 1987;17:17–21.
5. Rapoport DM, inventor; New York University, assignee. Method and apparatus for the treatment of obstructive sleep apnea. US patent 5,065,756. November 19, 1991.
6. Sullivan CE. ResMed origins. Available at: www.resmed.com/us/dam/documents/articles/resmed-origins.pdf. Accessed January 29, 2016.
7. Sanders MH, Kern NB, Stiller RA, et al. CPAP therapy via oronasal mask for obstructive sleep apnea. Chest 1994;106(3):774–9.
8. Prosise GL, Berry RB. Oral-nasal continuous positive airway pressure as a treatment for obstructive sleep apnea. Chest 1994;106:180–6.
9. Anderson FE, Kingshott RN, Taylor DR, et al. A randomized crossover efficacy trial of oral CPAP (Oracle) compared with nasal CPAP in the management of obstructive sleep apnea. Sleep 2003;26:721–6.
10. Axe JR, Behbehani K, Burk JR, et al, inventors; Board of Regents, The University of Texas System, assignee. Method and apparatus for controlling sleep disorder breathing. US patent 5,203,343. April 30, 1993.
11. Servidio JL, Tucker RF, inventors; Healthdyne, Inc, Marietta, GA, assignee. Nasal positive pressure device. US patent 5,117,819. July 2, 1992.
12. Gay P, Weaver T, Loube D, et al, Positive Airway Pressure Task Force, Standards of Practice Committee, American Academy of Sleep Medicine. Evaluation of positive airway pressure treatment for sleep related breathing disorders in adults. Sleep 2006; 29:381–401.
13. Pressman MR, Peterson DD, Meyer TJ, et al. Ramp abuse. A novel form of patient noncompliance to administration of nasal continuous positive airway pressure for treatment of obstructive sleep apnea. Am J Respir Crit Care Med 1995;151: 1632–4.
14. Ayappa I, Norman RG, Whiting D, et al. Irregular respiration as a marker of wakefulness during titration of CPAP. Sleep 2009;32:99–104.
15. Rapoport DM, Norman RG, inventors; New York University, New York, NY, assigned. Positive airway pressure system and method for treatment of sleeping disorder in patient. US patent 6,988,994. January 24, 2006.
16. Dungan GC II, Marshall NS, Hoyos CM, et al. A randomized crossover trial of the effect of a novel method of pressure control (SensAwake) in automatic continuous positive airway pressure therapy to treat sleep disordered breathing. J Clin Sleep Med 2011;7:261–7.
17. Sanders MH, Zdrojkowski RJ, inventors; Respironics, Inc, Murrysville, PA, assignee. Method and apparatus for maintaining airway patency to treat sleep apnea and other disorders. US patent 5,148,802. September 22, 1992.
18. Sanders MH, Zdrojkowski RJ, inventors; Respironics, Inc, Murrysville, PA, assignee. Breathing gas delivery method and apparatus. US patent 5,433,193. July 18, 1995.
19. Sanders MH, Kern N. Obstructive sleep apnea treated by independently adjusted inspiratory and expiratory positive airway pressures via nasal mask. Physiologic and clinical implications. Chest 1990;98:317–24.
20. Robertson PL, Roloff DW. Chronic respiratory failure in limb-girdle muscular dystrophy: successful long-term therapy with nasal bilevel positive airway pressure. Pediatr Neurol 1994;10:328–31.
21. Estes MC, Fiore JH, inventors; Respironics Inc, assignee. Method and apparatus for providing proportional positive airway pressure to treat sleep

disordered breathing. US patent 5,535,738. July 16, 1996.

22. Nilius G, Happel A, Domanski U, et al. Pressure-relief continuous positive airway pressure vs constant continuous positive airway pressure: a comparison of efficacy and compliance. Chest 2006;130:1018–24.

23. Masdeu MJ, Patel AV, Seelall V, et al. The supraglottic effect of a reduction in expiratory mask pressure during continuous positive airway pressure. Sleep 2012;35:263–72.

24. Smith I, Lasserson TJ. Pressure modification for improving usage of continuous positive airway pressure machines in adults with obstructive sleep apnoea. Cochrane Database Syst Rev 2009;(4): CD003531.

25. Bassin DJ, inventor; ResMed Limited, New South Wales, Australia, assignee. Methods for providing expiratory pressure relief in positive airway pressure therapy. US patent 7,866,318. January 11, 2011.

26. Bassin DJ, inventor; ResMed Limited, New South Wales, Australia, assignee. Methods for providing expiratory pressure relief in positive airway pressure therapy. US patent 8,899,231. December 2, 2014.

27. Berry RB, Parish JM, Hartse KM. The use of auto-titrating continuous positive airway pressure for treatment of adult obstructive sleep apnea. An American Academy of Sleep Medicine review. Sleep 2002;25:148–73.

28. Berthon-Jones M, Farrugia SP, inventors; ResMed Limited, North Ryde, Australia, assignee. Administration of CPAP treatment pressure in presence of apnea. US patent 6,367,474. April 9, 2002.

29. Sullivan CE, Lynch C, inventors; ResCare Limited, North Ryde, Australia, assignee. Device and method for monitoring breathing during sleep, control of CPAP treatment, and preventing of apnea. US patent 5,245,995. September 21, 1993.

30. Axe JR, Bebehani K, Burk JR, et al, inventors; Respironics Inc, Murrysville, PA, assignee. Method and apparatus for controlling sleep disorder breathing. US patent 5,458,137. October 17, 1995.

31. Alder M, Farrugia SP, Somaiya C, et al, inventors; ResMed Limited, assignee. Computer controlled CPAP system with snore detection. US patent 8,365,729. February 5, 2013.

32. Gradon LG, Whiting DR, Gerred AG, et al, inventors; Fisher & Paykel Healthcare Limited, Auckland, NZ, assignee. Autotitrating method and apparatus. US patent 7,882,834. February 8, 2011.

33. Ayappa I, Norman RG, Hosselet JJ, et al. Relative occurrence of flow limitation and snoring during continuous positive airway pressure titration. Chest 1998;114:685–90.

34. Luisada A. The internal pneumocardiogram. Am Heart J 1942;23:676–91.

35. Morrell MJ, Badr MS, Harms CA, et al. The assessment of upper airway patency during apnea using cardiogenic oscillations in the airflow signal. Sleep 1995;18:651–8.

36. Ayappa I, Norman RG, Rapoport DM. Cardiogenic oscillations on the airflow signal during continuous positive airway pressure as a marker of central apnea. Chest 1999;116:660–6.

37. Berthon-Jones M, inventor; ResMed Limited, North Ryde, Australia, assignee. Detection of apnea and obstruction of the airway in the respiratory system. US patent 5,704,345. January 6, 1998.

38. Rapport [sic] DM, Norman RG, inventors; New York University School of Medicine, assignee. Method and apparatus for optimizing controlled positive airway pressure using the detection of cardiogenic oscillations. US patent 6,739,335. May 25, 2004.

39. Berthon-Jones M, inventor; ResMed Limited, assignee. Determination of patency of the airway. US patent 7,320,320. January 22, 2008.

40. DuBois AB, Brody AW, Lewis DH, et al. Oscillation mechanics of lungs and chest in man. J Appl Physiol 1956;8:587–94.

41. Miller RD, Hyatt RE. Obstructing lesions of the larynx and trachea: clinical and physiologic characteristics. Mayo Clin Proc 1969;44:145–61.

42. Abramson AL, Goldstein MN, Stenzler A, et al. The use of the tidal breathing flow volume loop in laryngotracheal disease of neonates and infants. Laryngoscope 1982;92:922–6.

43. Condos R, Norman RG, Krishnasamy I, et al. Flow limitation as a noninvasive assessment of residual upper-airway resistance during continuous positive airway pressure therapy of obstructive sleep apnea. Am J Respir Crit Care Med 1994;150:475–80.

44. Sériès F, Marc I. Accuracy of breath-by-breath analysis of flow-volume loop in identifying sleep-induced flow-limited breathing cycles in sleep apnoea-hypopnoea syndrome. Clin Sci (Lond) 1995;88: 707–12.

45. Rapoport DM, inventor; New York University, assignee. Method and apparatus for continuous positive airway pressure for treating obstructive sleep apnea. US patent 5,335,654. August 9, 1994.

46. Rapoport DM, Norman RG, inventors; New York University, assignee. Method and apparatus for optimizing the continuous positive airway pressure for treating obstructive sleep apnea. US patent 5,490,502. February 13, 1996.

47. Matthews G, Kane MT, Duff WK, et al, inventors; RIC Investments, LLC, assignee. Auto-titration pressure support system and method of using same. US patent 7,827,988. November 9, 2010.

48. Javaheri S, Dempsey JA. Central sleep apnea. Compr Physiol 2013;3:141–63.

49. Javaheri S, Brown L, Randerath W. Positive airway pressure therapy with adaptive servo-ventilation

(Part 1: operational algorithms). Chest 2014;146: 514–23.

50. Berthon-Jones M, inventor; ResMed, Ltd, assignee. Ventilatory assistance for treatment of cardiac failure and Cheyne-Stokes breathing. US patent 6,532,959. March 18, 2003.

51. Teschler H, Dohring J, Wang YM, et al. Adaptive pressure support servo-ventilation: a novel treatment for Cheyne-Stokes respiration in heart failure. Am J Respir Crit Care Med 2001;164:614–9.

52. Brown S. Adaptive servo-ventilation using the ResMed VPAP adapt SV. Sleep Diagn Ther 2007;2: 20–2.

53. Pépin J-L, Chouri-Pontarollo N, Tamisier R, et al. Cheyne-Stokes respiration with central sleep apnoea in chronic heart failure: proposals for a diagnostic and therapeutic strategy. Sleep Med Rev 2006;10:33–47.

54. Cowie MR, Woehrle H, Wegscheider K, et al. Adaptive servo-ventilation for central sleep apnea in systolic heart failure. N Engl J Med 2015;373: 1095–105.

55. Hill PD, inventor; Respironics, Inc, assignee. Method and apparatus for providing variable positive airway pressure. US patent 6,752,151. June 22, 2004.

56. Zdrojkowski RJ, Estes M, inventors; Respironics, Inc, assignee. Breathing gas delivery method and apparatus. US patent 5,803,065. September 8, 1998.

57. Dedrick DL, Brown LK, Doggett JW, et al. Volume assured pressure support in adults with severe obstructive sleep apnea. Chest 2000;118:265S.

58. Hill PD, Kissel MH, Frank J, inventors; Respironics, Inc, assignee. Average volume ventilation. US patent 6,920,875. July 26, 2005.

59. Hill PD, Kissel MH, Frank J, et al, inventors; Average volume ventilation. US patent 7,011,091. March 14, 2006.

60. Murphy PB, Davidson C, Hind MD, et al. Volume targeted versus pressure support non-invasive ventilation in patients with super obesity and chronic respiratory failure: a randomised controlled trial. Thorax 2012;67:727–34.

61. Briones Claudett KH, Briones Claudett M, Chung Sang Wong M, et al. Noninvasive mechanical ventilation with average volume assured pressure support (AVAPS) in patients with chronic obstructive pulmonary disease and hypercapnic encephalopathy. BMC Pulm Med 2013;13:12.

62. Ambrogio C, Lowman X, Kuo M, et al. Sleep and non-invasive ventilation in patients with chronic respiratory insufficiency. Intensive Care Med 2009;35: 306–13.

63. Storre JH, Seuthe B, Fiechter R, et al. Average volume-assured pressure support in obesity hypoventilation: a randomized crossover trial. Chest 2006;130:815–21.

64. Janssens JP, Metzger M, Sforza E. Impact of volume targeting on efficacy of bi-level non-invasive ventilation and sleep in obesity-hypoventilation. Respir Med 2009;103:165–72.

65. Pluym M, Kabir AW, Gohar A. The use of volume-assured pressure support noninvasive ventilation in acute and chronic respiratory failure: a practical guide and literature review. Hosp Pract 1995; 2015(43):299–307.

66. Berthon-Jones M, inventor; Resmed [sic] Limited, North Ryde, Australia, assignee. Assisted ventilation to match patient respiratory need. US patent 6,532,957. March 18, 2003.

67. Bassin DJ, inventor; ResMed Limited, assignee. Methods and apparatus for varying the back-up rate for a ventilator. US patent 8,448,640. May 28, 2013.

68. ResMed Inc. Stellar series. Available at: https://www.resmed.com/us/dam/documents/products/machine/stellar-3/clinical-guide/248905_stellar-100-150_clinical-guide_amer_eng.pdf. Accessed August 18, 2017.

69. Berthon-Jones M, Bateman P, Bassin D, Malouf G, inventors; ResMed Limited, assignee. Determining suitable ventilator settings for patients with alveolar hypoventilation during sleep. US patent 8,544,467. October 1, 2013.

70. Kelly JL, Jaye J, Pickersgill RE, et al. Randomized trial of 'intelligent' autotitrating ventilation versus standard pressure support non-invasive ventilation: impact on adherence and physiological outcomes. Respirology 2014;19:596–603.

71. Oscroft NS, Chadwick R, Davies MG, et al. Volume assured versus pressure preset non-invasive ventilation for compensated ventilatory failure in COPD. Respir Med 2014;108:1508–15.

72. Johnson KG, Johnson DC. Treatment of sleep-disordered breathing with positive airway pressure devices: technology update. Med Devices (Auckl) 2015;8:425–37.

73. Brown LK. Autotitrating CPAP: how shall we judge safety and efficacy of a "black box"? Chest 2006; 130:312–4.

74. Schwab RJ, Badr SM, Epstein LJ, et al. An Official American Thoracic Society Statement: continuous positive airway pressure adherence tracking systems. The optimal monitoring strategies and outcome measures in adults. Am J Respir Crit Care Med 2013;188:613–20.

# Testing the Performance of Positive Airway Pressure Generators
## From Bench to Bedside

Kaixian Zhu, PhD[a],*, Claire Colas des Francs, MD[b],
Amélie Sagniez, MSc[a], Pierre Escourrou, MD, PhD[b]

### KEYWORDS

• Bench evaluations • Clinical evaluations • PAP treatment • Sleep disordered breathing

### KEY POINTS

• Positive airway pressure (PAP) devices use different proprietary algorithms for sleep-disordered breathing event detection and response.
• Clinical evaluations allow measuring long-term treatment efficacy, but have limitations such as patient variability and high cost.
• Bench studies are necessary to evaluate devices in predefined conditions for understanding algorithms of detection and treatment of disordered breathing events.
• Combining results of bench tests and clinical studies is essential to improve the management of patients with PAP treatment.

## INTRODUCTION

The clinician applying a positive airway pressure (PAP) treatment to a patient needs to obtain the following information:

1. Is the treatment safe for the overall condition of the patient?
2. Is the treatment efficient on the disease abnormalities?
3. Is the treatment adherence adequate for obtaining the best outcomes?
4. Is there any side effect at the interface (leaks) or inadequate patient–device interaction (such as arousals linked to the device functioning) that may impair treatment efficacy or tolerance?

Newer PAP generators can track adherence, hours of use, mask or mouth leak, and residual apnea–hypopnea index (AHI). Such data seem very useful to follow chronic disease outcomes. However, there are no standard for recording adherence data, scoring flow signals, or measuring leak, or for how clinicians should use these data.

According to the US Food and Drug Administration and the European Community regulations, PAP generators are class II devices, which may carry risks to the patient. Marketing approval for positive airway generators in the United States follows the simplified 510(k) procedure in which a device only require that clinical studies demonstrate equivalent ability to suppress sleep-disordered breathing (SDB) events in comparison with a previously approved apparatus.[1] This historical comparison may go back to devices manufactured many years before the newly sold device,

Disclosure Statement: The authors have nothing to disclose.
[a] Centre Explor, Air Liquide Healthcare, 28 rue d'Arcueil, Gentilly 94250, France; [b] Sleep Disorders Center, AP-HP Antoine-Béclère Hospital, 157 rue de la Porte de Trivaux, Clamart 92140, France
* Corresponding author.
E-mail address: kaixian.zhu@gmail.com

incorporating very different technology. The European directives also have a requirement for approving family of devices on clinical data, which may be "published and/or unpublished reports on other clinical experience of either the device in question or a similar device for which equivalence to the device in question can be demonstrated."[2]

Indeed, for these devices there is no required thorough certification process similar to what is required for any new drug. Because clinical studies are long and costly, it is common practice to introduce a new product to the market without specific clinical evaluation.

The PAP generators are in their principle, simple devices based on a blower that takes room air and generates airflow through flexible tubing at a pre-set pressure that is determined at the mask interface with the patient. Continuous PAP (CPAP) devices are used in most sleep apnea patients in the long term, but the settings are usually titrated during several nights at home, using an auto-adjusting PAP (APAP) because manual titration in the sleep laboratory is costly and suffers long waiting lists. Because algorithms often are not disclosed, this technology is often seen as a "black box" that collects and analyses data to detect breathing abnormalities and provide a treatment supposedly adapted to the patient condition.[3]

Given that APAP are a relatively new technology, there are no generally accepted criteria for defining the optimum method of modifying the mask pressure in response to breathing events so that devices provide different results when subjected to the same breathing pattern. Therefore, the individual demonstration of their efficacy is very relevant. This evaluation cannot rely on symptoms, because controlled trials have demonstrated a noticeable placebo effect[4,5] and would require costly sleep laboratory studies. An alternative approach is the use of bench testing to challenge each device by events as close as possible to patients breathing events.

PAP usages seem to be reliably determined from device-reported compliance data, but a definitive accuracy study has not been published. The residual events (apnea or hypopnea) and leak data are not as easy to interpret and the definitions of these parameters differ among PAP manufacturers.[6]

Any observed difference in residual AHI between bench values and device-reported ones bear considerable clinical implications, because the current follow-up of patient often relies on device-reported residual AHI, which may be very different from actual patient values.[7–12]

It is the aim of this paper to describe this methodology and investigate how bench results can help clinicians in evaluating the treatment efficacy of PAP devices and the reliability of device-reported data.

## BENCH TESTING OF DYNAMIC PERFORMANCE OF POSITIVE AIRWAY PRESSURE DEVICES
### Pressure Stability and Effects of Leaks

PAP devices should maintain a stable positive pressure or provide a bilevel pressure in the airway during respiratory cycles with the presence of normal pressure swings from breathing and deviations in pressure caused by leaks. Therefore, these devices should offer both static and dynamic pressure stability, that is, to compensate pressure swing during each respiratory cycle. For older PAP devices, airway pressure significantly varied during the respiratory cycle, especially when the breathing flow rate was high.[13,14] Bench studies showed a higher dynamic pressure stability in bilevel PAP devices than in CPAPs owing to different technologies applied in the blowers.[13,14] Recent devices can measure the pressure loss in the patient's tubing and adjust the pressure in dynamic conditions.[15]

PAP devices can also compensate for up to a certain level of leaks.[16] **Fig. 1** shows an example of airway pressure changes of 2 CPAP devices subjected to different levels of leak. The pressure stability with leaks has significant impacts on treatment efficacy. Bench studies on APAPs demonstrated that air leaks may affect the responses of devices and cause airway pressure to significantly

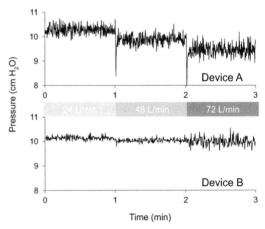

Fig. 1. Airway pressure change of 2 continuous positive airway pressure (CPAP) devices subjected to 3 levels of leak: 24, 48, and 72 L/min calibrated at 10 cm H$_2$O. The pressure of CPAP devices were set at 10 cm H$_2$O. Differences between these 2 devices are significant in pressure stability and in the capacity of leak compensation.

drop below a set pressure.[17,18] Regarding bench studies on bilevel PAP, Mehta and colleagues[19] showed that leaking interfered with cycling, inverting I:E ratio, shortening expiratory time thus reducing delivered tidal volume, and suggested adjusting ventilator settings to avoid patient–ventilator asynchrony. Borel and colleagues[20] demonstrated that patient's tidal volume was significantly reduced because of leaks higher than 40 L/min, which led to reduced capacity of achieving and maintaining inspiratory pressure in bilevel devices. Bench studies also showed that increased patient's work of breathing could result from leaking[15] or pressure swings during breathing cycles.[14]

## Pressure Compensation for Altitude Change

Changes in altitude do not significantly alter absolute pressure requirement in patients with obstructive sleep apnea (OSA) treatment.[21] However, a bench evaluation performed by Fromm and colleagues[22] demonstrated that altitude exposure could significantly alter the delivered pressure of PAP devices. When the altitude increased, fan speed of the blower of PAP devices needed to increase to maintain the set pressure.[22,23] Many devices on the market can automatically adjust to altitude.[23] A recent study of bench simulation confirmed that CPAP devices equipped with a pressure sensor were more reliable in maintaining the pressure level regardless of altitude and ambient pressure changes.[24]

## BENCH TESTING OF ALGORITHMS OF AUTO-ADJUSTING POSITIVE AIRWAY PRESSURE DEVICES
### Principles of Bench Models

Bench studies have been proposed to evaluate the responses of APAP devices in various but controlled conditions, such as the presence of predefined SDB patterns with[17,18,25] and without nonintentional leaks.[26–33] In the literature, bench models for evaluating APAP devices can be divided into 2 main categories according to the response of the model to tested devices: the systems that do not react to changes in airway pressure (open loop) and those that take into account pressure changes administrated by the tested devices (closed loop). **Table 1** shows the principles of these bench models in the literature.

The first open-loop bench model for APAP evaluation was reported by Farré and colleagues.[17] This model principally consisted of a breathing simulator that was able to reproduce breathing flow signals recorded from actual patients. Snoring and leakage could also be simulated with the

model. During the test, the airway pressure and flow signals were acquired and these signals allowed further analysis of the responses of the tested device, which was subjected to predefined breathing patterns. A similar model was developed by Lofaso and colleagues[27] for evaluating flow limitation detection by APAP devices. Note that no mechanical obstruction was simulated in either model, and obstructive breathing events were simulated at the "flow generator" level instead of the "upper airway."

Considering this inconvenient, Rigau and colleagues[25] improved the model of Farré and colleagues by adding a servo-controlled valve, which allowed the simulation of obstructive events by imposing the mechanical impedance of the upper airway. According to the authors, this valve was controlled in a closed loop driven by pressure in the airway. The airway obstruction could thus respond to the APAP-administrated airway pressure, whereas the control law of the valve was not detailed in the publication. Identical to the previous model, the improved model was able to reproduce any flow waveforms recorded in patients. This model was recently updated by Isetta and colleagues[33] and the library of patients' SDB events was enriched. However, it should be highlighted that recorded patient's flow signals for driving the flow generator were already the consequences of the combination of inspiratory efforts and upper airway obstructions. It is, thus, difficult to determine the contribution of each separate abnormality from the resultant flow signal alone. Therefore, the interaction between the tested APAP device and the servo-controlled valve was limited by the control law and the algorithm of the bench model.

Instead of a servo-controlled valve, a "Starling resistor" consisting of a collapsible tube in a sealed chamber was used to simulate the human upper airway.[18,26,28–30,32,34] The opening of the tube was adjusted by changing the transmural pressure applied on the tube. This mechanical element allowed the bench model to work in a closed loop by adapting the opening of the tube precisely in response to the tested APAP device. However, the characteristics of the breathing flow waveform, which may influence the reaction of APAP devices, were difficult to reproduce precisely with a Starling resistor.

In addition to the upper airway, the lung model is important especially for evaluating ventilators in diseased lung conditions. Among the bench models previously mentioned, 3 types of lung models were applied: Training and Test Lung (Michigan Instruments, Grand Rapids, MI; "Michigan lung"),[18,26–28] servo-controlled

**Table 1**
**Bench model for auto-adjusting positive airway pressure and adaptive servo-ventilation evaluations**

| Related Publications | Lung Model | Upper Airway Model | Control |
|---|---|---|---|
| Farré et al,[17] 2002 | Computer-controlled pump | N/A | Open-loop control The pump was driven by patient's signal |
| Abdenbi et al,[26] 2004 | "Michigan" test lung | Starling resistor | Closed-loop control Test lung generated sinusoidal flow |
| Coller et al,[18] 2005 | "Michigan" test lung | Starling resistor; adjusted by a syringe | Closed-loop control Test lung generated sinusoidal flow |
| Lofaso et al,[27] 2006 | "Michigan" test lung | N/A | Open-loop control Test lung was driven by a flow generator that regulated by a servo-controlled valve |
| Rigau et al,[26] 2006; Isetta et al,[31] 2015; Isetta et al,[33] 2016 | Computer-controlled pump | Servo-controlled valve | Closed-loop control at the upper airway |
| Hirose et al,[28] 2008 | "Michigan" test lung | Starling resistor | Closed-loop control Additional upstream resistance was added in the upper airway |
| Zhu et al,[34] 2013 | Computer-controlled pump with respiratory balloon | Starling resistor | Closed-loop control |
| Netzel et al,[29] 2014 | "Hamburg" active lung model | Starling resistor | Closed-loop control |
| Zhu et al,[30] 2015; Zhu et al,[32] 2016 | ASL 5000 | Starling resistor | Closed-loop control |

*Abbreviation:* N/A, not applicable.

pump,[17,25,31,33] and sophisticated active test lung models.[29,30,32] The Michigan test lung was a mechanical model consisting of 2 bellows. One bellow (master bellow) was connected to a driving ventilator and simulated the activities of inspiratory muscles, and the second bellow (slave bellow) was driven by the master bellow and was connected to the tested PAP device. The lung properties such as intrathoracic airway resistance and compliance could be adjusted mechanically, for example, the system compliance was modified by manually changing the position of a spring on the bellow. This system was not designed for complex inspiratory effort simulations.

The computer-driven piston was able to replicate the breathing waveform with high accuracy, and the response of PAP device subjected to specific breathing patterns could be analyzed. However, the system worked in an open loop and did not react to administrated pressure of tested PAP devices owing to limited mechanical

properties of the artificial lung. As a solution, a respiratory balloon could be added in parallel to the flow generator to provide compliance.[34] In addition, sophisticated active lung models such as ASL 5000 (IngMar Medical, Pittsburgh, PA) that simulates mechanical lung properties and inspiratory efforts were used for bench evaluations of PAP devices.[29,30] This allowed testing PAP devices in a closed loop at the lung level. **Fig. 2** gives an example of bench model for APAP device evaluations.

### Bench Evaluations of Positive Airway Pressure Devices

#### Auto-adjusting positive airway pressure
APAP devices on the market perform differently on bench tests.[17,30] This may result from difference in the algorithms for detection and/or response of the devices. To understand the algorithms of devices, bench-simulated breathing

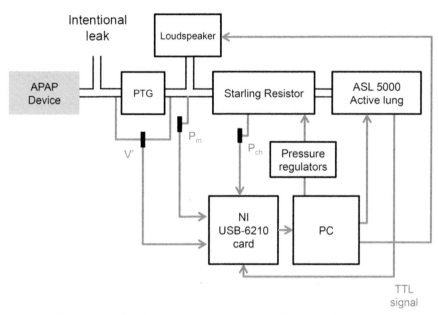

**Fig. 2.** An example of bench model with upper airway simulation for auto-adjusting positive airway pressure (APAP) evaluation. Intentional leak, 24 L/min calibrated at 10 cm $H_2O$; Pch, measured chamber pressure of the Starling resistor; Pm, measured mask pressure; PTG, pneumotachograph; TTL, transistor-transistor logic; V′, measured mask flow. (*From* Zhu K, Roisman G, Aouf S, et al. All APAPs are not equivalent for the treatment of sleep disordered breathing: a bench evaluation of eleven commercially available devices. J Clin Sleep Med 2015;11(7):726; with permission.)

sequences with repetitive single-type SDB events allowed testing detection and reaction to specific SDB events.[17,29,30] Results showed a large variability between devices in the capacity of SDB event detection, which could be caused by the detection techniques used by each device. For example, some devices considered cardiac oscillations as a surrogate of an open upper airway,[23,30] whereas the sensitivity of cardiac oscillation was reported as only 60% for central apnea diagnosis.[35] In contrast, the forced oscillation technique applied by some devices was considered more mature and reliable because this technique was widely used for measuring the airway impedance in lung function tests.[36] The detection of SDB events was also influenced by the definitions applied by device manufacturers, such as airflow amplitude, event duration, and acoustic vibrations, and so on, which are often at variance with the American Academy of Sleep Medicine guidelines.[37,38] In addition to SDB event detection, the protocols for increasing and decreasing pressure also differed between device manufacturers.[23,30]

Test protocols of repetitive single-type SDB events had limitations, because such controlled, regular breathing flow rarely occurred in real clinical conditions. A variety of characteristics and phenotypes exist not only between patients, but

also occur within the same subject during different sleep stages and body positions. New APAP devices were equipped with advanced algorithms to recognize long sequences of events from measured patient's flow, and the pressure response of the device to such events could be different to a single isolated event. For example, repetitive apneas that persisted at high PAP were considered as "non-responding" events by some devices such as the RemStar APAP devices (Philips Respironics, Murrysville, PA). The administrated pressure thus decreased when the device was subjected to periodic breathing.[32] To approach clinical and complex conditions, 2 recent bench studies have simulated patient's full-night sleep breathing scenarios including a variety of SDB patterns: Zhu and colleagues[30] evaluated 11 APAP devices on a 5.75-hour scenario including the simulated breathing patterns of 4 sleep cycles. They found that only 5 devices obtained a residual obstructive AHI of less than 5 per hour. Isetta and colleagues[33] simulated a typical night of sleep of a female patient with OSA and tested 10 APAP devices. As a result, only 3 devices were able to overcome flow limitations and 5 devices presented a residual AHI of less than 5 per hour.

In addition, a recent bench study questioned the impact of pressure relief modes on CPAP treatment efficacy.[32] The pressure relief modes are aimed at improving patients' comfort during CPAP treatment. The results of the bench study showed that the CPAP efficacy could be attenuated if the set pressure was not adjusted for, at the time of introduction of pressure relief modes, and suggested enabling such features before initial pressure titration.

In addition, new PAP devices provide treatment reports on which the device-estimated residual AHI is shown. The accuracy of this index was questioned in one bench study.[30] As a result, 7 devices out of 11 identified AHI with an accuracy of greater than 90%. Such differences could be explained by the different definitions of SDB events applied by device manufacturers, which obviously must differ from American Academy of Sleep Medicine rules for scoring respiratory events,[37,38] because they do not take into account oxygen desaturations and arousals to determine hypopneas, or total sleep time to compute an actual AHI.

### Bilevel positive airway pressure and adaptive servo-ventilation

Bilevel PAP device alternates the airway pressure during inspiration (inspiratory PAP) and expiration (expiratory PAP, EPAP). Note that bilevel PAP without backup rate (BiPAP, Philips Respironics) is indicated for patients with OSA who cannot tolerate a high level of pressure. The objective is to increase patient comfort and improve the treatment compliance.[39]

Bilevel PAP noninvasive ventilation with backup rate is aimed at improving gas exchange in hypercapnic patients with obstructive and central apneas and respiratory insufficiency caused by obstructive or restrictive lung diseases. In the literature, bench evaluations of bilevel devices focused on pressurization rate,[40] patient–ventilator interactions such as triggering and cycling,[41,42] the effect of condensate in the tubing,[43] and the accuracy of estimations of tidal volume and leakage.[44–47] Different from the bench models previously mentioned for APAPs, most benches for bilevel PAP evaluation did not use a variable upper airway resistance, although occurrence of obstructive events are frequent in patients treated by such devices. In addition, a recent review of studies on bilevel PAP devices[48] highlighted several limitations: unclear impacts of different lung models applied, inconsistent settings of tested devices, different terminology, and lack of standard criteria for measurement.

Adaptive servo-ventilation is a specific bilevel PAP that provides variable pressure support, that is, the difference between inspiratory PAP and EPAP. New devices use similar algorithms to APAP for adjusting the EPAP to overcome obstructive SDB patterns.[49] The device is indicated for treating patients with central and mixed apneas and periodic breathing such as Cheyne-Stokes breathing. Zhu and colleagues[34] reported a bench evaluation of 3 adaptive servo-ventilation devices, of which 2 devices had autotitrated EPAP. The 3 tested devices eliminated all bench-simulated central apneas of Cheyne-Stokes breathing, and these events were transformed to hypopneas. The obstructive events were treated differently between devices. For the adaptive servo-ventilation with constant EPAP (AutoSet CS, Resmed [San Diego, CA], is similar to VPAP Adapt available in the US market), the obstructive events were partially cleared with high-level pressure support despite of a low EPAP value of 4 cm $H_2O$. Autotriggering was also observed in this device during normal breathing. The accuracy of the device-estimated AHI depended on initial settings of devices. Advantages and limitations of bench tests are summarized in **Table 2**.

## WHAT CAN WE LEARN FROM CLINICAL EVALUATIONS?

Compared with bench evaluations, clinical tests allow access to long-term safety evaluations and measurement of associated physiologic parameters (see **Table 2**). However, these studies are often limited by small numbers of patients, short follow-up, and limited compliance. Sometimes, well-conducted studies did not reflect clinical practice because patients with hypnotic treatment or significant comorbidities such as insomnia or chronic obstructive pulmonary disease were excluded, limiting the generalization of findings to real patient populations.

### Treatment Efficacy of Auto-adjusting Positive Airway Pressure Devices

The clinical efficacy of APAP has been questioned by some studies showing a large residual AHI with some devices.[50] Early studies that attempted to explore PAP device effectiveness were based on the capacity of normalizing the AHI manually scored with a polysomnography (PSG). One limitation is that evaluations were performed during the titration night and did not reflect long-term use of treatment. The poor performances of some devices may explain the observation of a poorer control of blood pressure with APAP, which was associated with a higher residual AHI.[51] More recent studies have also underlined a less beneficial effect of APAP than CPAP on autonomic nervous system activation measurements, such as

**Table 2**
**Advantages and limitations of bench and clinical evaluations**

|  | Advantages | Limitations |
|---|---|---|
| Bench evaluation | • Reproducibility of test conditions<br>• Predefined specific test conditions<br>• Results of specific needs (eg, delay of response to an event; pressure rising time)<br>• Objectivity<br>• Reliability<br>• Didactic methods and results<br>• Possibility to measure the dynamic performances and to understand the algorithms<br>• Low cost<br>• Study duration relatively short | • Short-term performance of PAP devices; impossible to deduce long-term therapeutic effects<br>• Impossible to get subjective feedback from patients<br>• Simulated patient characteristics are limited; some physiologic conditions are not taken into account (eg, neurologic loop)<br>• Consequence of some physiologic parameters cannot be evaluated (eg, $SpO_2$) |
| Clinical evaluation | • Data available for long-term therapeutic effects<br>• Unique way to measure the compliance of patient<br>• Get patient's subjective treatment feedback directly<br>• Measurement of physiologic parameters ($SpO_2$, arousals, etc.)<br>• Long-term safety evaluation | • Intrapatient and interpatient variability; a large number of subjects are needed to get reliable results<br>• Difficulty to get strictly identical conditions (impossible to predict identical SDB events in patients of OSA)<br>• Difficulty to measure the dynamic performance of devices<br>• Disturbing factors for clinical evaluation such as medication and alcohol<br>• High cost<br>• Long durations of studies |

*Abbreviations:* OSA, obstructive sleep apnea; PAP, positive airway pressure; SDB, sleep disordered breathing.

heart rate variability[52,53] or pulse wave amplitude.[12] APAP devices have also been questioned in some studies on sleep disturbances linked to arousals seemingly secondary to rapid pressure increases in reaction to SDB events.[54]

A recent metaanalysis showed that the symptomatic effects of treatment are similar between APAP and CPAP.[55] Meurice and colleagues,[50] in 2007, were the first to compare APAP and CPAP devices in a long-term protocol in 83 patients with severe sleep apnea–hypopnea syndrome. Patients were randomly allocated to 1 of 5 different groups: fixed CPAP after titration performed in the laboratory and the 4 other groups used different APAP machines. No difference was demonstrated in average device effectiveness based on PSG parameters between the 5 groups; nevertheless, in some individuals the residual AHI remained elevated particularly for 2 devices (SomnoSmart, Weinmann [Hamburg, Germany] and Pv10i, Breas [Mölnlycke, Sweden]). Furthermore, APAP was shown in some patients to be less effective than fixed pressure on manually scored PSG, even if the average

residual AHI given by the device seemed to be correct.

These findings have been confirmed by bench studies, which have found inadequate treatment of certain hypopneas and delayed response in correcting apneas[17,26] and other clinical studies reporting a high proportion of undertreated patients on APAP.[56,57]

## Reliability of Device-Reported Apnea–Hypopnea Index

Reports of residual events obtained by the devices have also been questioned by some authors.[7–11,58] Few studies have documented the accuracy of event detection algorithms.

Denotti and colleagues[8] investigated whether deficiencies of APAP resulted from failures to detect or to respond to airway obstruction. In this study, airflow was measured both at nasal mask and directly from APAP devices (Auto-Set T, Resmed) and both signals were recorded on PSG. AHIs at these 2 sites were compared with device-estimated AHI in the device reports. The authors found that nasal flow AHI was in agreement with APAP flow AHI, although agreement was lower with device-estimated AHI. There was a trend for APAP to underestimate the AHI at higher actual value and overestimate it at lower values. Failure in OSA detection resulted in risks of inadequate treatment. The results suggested that the built-in detection algorithm might result in incorrect estimation of residual AHI in some patients with OSAs and alert clinicians to interpret APAP reports with caution.

Berry and colleagues[58] compared the automatic event detection (AED) of SDB events of a PAP device (REMstar Auto M-Series, Philips Respironics) with manual scoring of PSG during PAP treatment. The agreement for apnea detection was better than hypopnea. An event-by-event analysis showed that the AED algorithm had a sensitivity of 0.58 and a specificity of 0.98, and an AED-AHI greater than 10 events per hour had a sensitivity of 0.58 and a specificity of 0.94. Thus, AED algorithms are reliable when the residual AHI is low. An AED-AHI of less than 10 events per hour indicates good treatment efficacy. The authors also suggested coupling the current algorithm with oximetry to better estimate the residual AHI and to detect periods of hypoxemia owing to hypoventilation.

Similar results were obtained for this particular device on a bench study at a much lower cost, showing a good control of the apnea, although hypopnea only partly reversed. Reported residual AHI did not significantly differ from the bench value indicating a good performance of the detection algorithm.[30]

Underestimated AHIs in some APAP devices were observed in bench studies with short treatment durations (95 minutes), although the difference in AHI was not significant between device report and bench when treatment duration is long (5.75 hours).[30] Device-reported AHI could be affected by leaks, but to our knowledge no bench study has specifically addressed this point.

## Compliance with Auto-adjusting Positive Airway Pressure Treatment

Long-term compliance with PAP treatment cannot be predicted on the bench. One approach has been suggested by Netzel and colleagues[29] by computing an arbitrary performance scale on the bench test and comparing it with the mean compliance data obtained in a large sample of patients using this device. Nevertheless, this kind of relationship is necessarily linked to many other factors then the device itself: mask interface used, pressure settings, education, and care of the patients, which are difficult to control for.

## Pressure Relief Features

Pressure relief features are developed to overcome patient difficulty of exhaling against a fixed pressure during fixed CPAP treatment and to improve the treatment adherence. However, for C-Flex, better adherence has not been consistently proven in clinical studies,[12,59–66] and the majority of studies reported similar adherence[59,61,66,67] and treatment efficacy[61] between CPAP with and without C-Flex. Adherence and similar treatment efficacy are not available in the literature for the other pressure relief features in CPAP devices.

Regarding APAP treatment with pressure relief features, Mulgrew and colleagues[68] found a nonsignificant trend of greater subjective comfort with C-Flex. Kushida and colleagues[69] reported identical treatment adherence and efficacy between A-Flex and conventional CPAP after either 3 or 6 months, but a higher AHI at the initiation phase. In a recent study, Chihara and colleagues[70] compared the adherence between conventional APAP, APAP with C-Flex, and APAP with A-Flex, and found a greater adherence in APAP with C-Flex. Of note, at the initiation of the studies of Kushida and colleagues and Chihara and colleagues, the APAP auto-titration was carried out with the activated pressure relief feature. However, the question rises concerning the risk of undertreating some patients, because the mean pressure is reduced by these "comfort modes," as shown on the bench, if pressure is not readjusted to a higher level.[32]

## Adaptive Servo-Ventilation in Patients with Severe Heart Failure

Another concern was recently raised by the safety issue of the Serve-HF study, where increased mortality was observed in patients with severe heart failure.[71] Because the reasons for this serious adverse event are not evident, it is worth questioning the performance of the device used which was Autoset CS2 (Resmed). This device has been shown to deliver a higher mean pressure on the bench compared with other devices and experienced asynchronies.[34] These mechanisms may have impaired further cardiac function with adverse consequences.

## Telemonitoring

Telemonitoring of PAP is now available from built-in GSM or WIFI transmission of device data. However, some health care providers rely on external devices placed on the tubing of the PAP device to analyze events and reports on compliance, residual indices and leaks; these systems clearly need a bench validation.[72] Furthermore, measuring and reporting the parameters from CPAP downloads are not standardized between manufacturers and not well-validated, so that the reports are not easily exportable to electronic medical records. Standardization is needed in this field.

## SUMMARY

PAP devices rely on different proprietary algorithms for SDB event detection and response. Most evaluations of such devices are based on clinical studies to test the clinical outcomes, the comfort and adherence of patients, and the impact on quality of life and long-term safety. Clinical studies have obvious limitations, such as patient variability, high cost, and long duration. As a complementary approach, bench studies provide an analysis of algorithms in predefined conditions, which allows understanding contradictory results observed in clinical studies. However, long-term treatment data and physiologic effects of PAP treatment cannot be assessed on the bench. It is important to understand the advantages and the limitations of both kinds of studies summarized in **Table 2**. In fact, clinical and bench studies are complementary. Combining results of bench tests and clinical studies is essential to improve the management of patients with PAP treatment.

## REFERENCES

1. The 510(k) program: evaluating substantial equivalence in premarket notifications [510(k)] - Guidance for Industry and Food and Drug Administration Staff. Available at: http://www.fda.gov/MedicalDevices/DeviceRegulationandGuidance/GuidanceDocuments/ucm404770.htm. Accessed December 19, 2014.
2. European Council. Directive 2007/47/EC. Available at: http://ec.europa.eu/consumers/sectors/medical-devices/files/revision_docs/2007-47-en_en.pdf. Accessed November 14, 2016.
3. Brown LK. Autotitrating CPAP: how shall we judge safety and efficacy of a "black box"? Chest 2006; 130(2):312–4.
4. Montserrat JM, Ferrer M, Hernandez L, et al. Effectiveness of CPAP treatment in daytime function in sleep apnea syndrome. Am J Respir Crit Care Med 2001;164(4):608–13.
5. Jenkinson C, Davies RJ, Mullins R, et al. Comparison of therapeutic and subtherapeutic nasal continuous positive airway pressure for obstructive sleep apnoea: a randomised prospective parallel trial. Lancet 1999;353(9170):2100–5.
6. Schwab RJ, Badr SM, Epstein LJ, et al. An official American Thoracic Society statement: continuous positive airway pressure adherence tracking systems. The optimal monitoring strategies and outcome measures in adults. Am J Respir Crit Care Med 2013;188(5):613–20.
7. Desai H, Patel A, Patel P, et al. Accuracy of autotitrating CPAP to estimate the residual apnea–hypopnea index in patients with obstructive sleep apnea on treatment with autotitrating CPAP. Sleep Breath 2009;13(4):383–90.
8. Denotti AL, Wong KKH, Dungan GC 2nd, et al. Residual sleep-disordered breathing during autotitrating continuous positive airway pressure therapy. Eur Respir J 2012;39(6):1391–7.
9. Ikeda Y, Kasai T, Kawana F, et al. Comparison between the apnea-hypopnea indices determined by the REMstar auto M series and those determined by standard in-laboratory polysomnography in patients with obstructive sleep apnea. Intern Med 2012;51(20):2877–85.
10. Cilli A, Uzun R, Bilge U. The accuracy of autotitrating CPAP-determined residual apnea–hypopnea index. Sleep Breath 2013;17(1):189–93.
11. Ueno K, Kasai T, Brewer G, et al. Evaluation of the apnea-hypopnea index determined by the S8 auto-CPAP, a continuous positive airway pressure device, in patients with obstructive sleep apnea-hypopnea syndrome. J Clin Sleep Med 2010;6(2):146–51.
12. Bakker JP, Campbell AJ, Neill AM. Pulse wave analysis in a pilot randomised controlled trial of auto-adjusting and continuous positive airway pressure for obstructive sleep apnoea. Sleep Breath 2011; 15(3):325–32.
13. Netzel N, Kirbas G, Matthys H, et al. Technical differences in various CPAP and BiLevel CPAP devices. Pneumologie 1997;51(Suppl 3):789–95 [in German].
14. Schäfer T, Vogelsang H. Pressure stability of nasal CPAP and bilevel devices. Somnologie 2002;6(2): 79–84.
15. Louis B, Leroux K, Boucherie M, et al. Pressure stability with CPAP devices: a bench evaluation. Sleep Med 2010;11(1):96–9.
16. Scala R. Bi-level home ventilators for non invasive positive pressure ventilation. Monaldi Arch Chest Dis 2004;61(4):213–21. Available at: http://www.monaldi-archives.org/index.php/macd/article/view/684. Accessed November 14, 2016.
17. Farré R, Montserrat JM, Rigau J, et al. Response of automatic continuous positive airway pressure devices to different sleep breathing patterns: a bench study. Am J Respir Crit Care Med 2002;166(4):469–73.
18. Coller D, Stanley D, Parthasarathy S. Effect of air leak on the performance of auto-PAP devices: a bench study. Sleep Breath 2005;9(4):167–75.

19. Mehta S, McCool FD, Hill NS. Leak compensation in positive pressure ventilators: a lung model study. Eur Respir J 2001;17(2):259–67.

20. Borel JC, Sabil A, Janssens J-P, et al. Intentional leaks in industrial masks have a significant impact on efficacy of bilevel noninvasive ventilation: a bench test study. Chest 2009;135(3):669–77.

21. Patz DS, Swihart B, White DP. CPAP pressure requirements for obstructive sleep apnea patients at varying altitudes. Sleep 2010;33(5):715–8.

22. Fromm J, Robert E, Varon J, et al. CPAP machine performance and altitude. Chest 1995;108(6):1577–80.

23. Johnson K, Johnson D. Treatment of sleep-disordered breathing with positive airway pressure devices: technology update. Med Devices Evid Res 2015;425. http://dx.doi.org/10.2147/MDER.S70062.

24. Sehlin M, Brändström H, Winsö O, et al. Simulated flying altitude and performance of continuous positive airway pressure devices. Aviat Space Environ Med 2014;85(11):1092–9.

25. Rigau J, Montserrat JM, Wöhrle H, et al. Bench model to simulate upper airway obstruction for analyzing automatic continuous positive airway pressure devices. Chest 2006;130(2):350–61.

26. Abdenbi F, Chambille B, Escourrou P. Bench testing of auto-adjusting positive airway pressure devices. Eur Respir J 2004;24(4):649–58.

27. Lofaso F, Desmarais G, Leroux K, et al. Bench evaluation of flow limitation detection by automated continuous positive airway pressure devices. Chest 2006;130(2):343–9.

28. Hirose M, Honda J, Sato E, et al. Bench study of auto-CPAP devices using a collapsible upper airway model with upstream resistance. Respir Physiol Neurobiol 2008;162(1):48–54.

29. Netzel T, Hein H, Hein Y. APAP device technology and correlation with patient compliance. Somnologie - Schlafforschung Schlafmed 2014;18(2):113–20.

30. Zhu K, Roisman G, Aouf S, et al. All APAPs are not equivalent for the treatment of sleep disordered breathing: a bench evaluation of eleven commercially available devices. J Clin Sleep Med 2015;11(7):725–34.

31. Isetta V, Navajas D, Montserrat JM, et al. Comparative assessment of several automatic CPAP devices' responses: a bench test study. ERJ Open Res 2015;1(1) [pii:00031-2015].

32. Zhu K, Aouf S, Roisman G, et al. Pressure-relief features of fixed and autotitrating continuous positive airway pressure may impair their efficacy: evaluation with a respiratory bench model. J Clin Sleep Med 2016;12(3):385–92.

33. Isetta V, Montserrat JM, Santano R, et al. Novel approach to simulate sleep apnea patients for evaluating positive pressure therapy devices. PLoS One 2016;11(3):e0151530.

34. Zhu K, Kharboutly H, Ma J, et al. Bench test evaluation of adaptive servoventilation devices for sleep apnea treatment. J Clin Sleep Med 2013;9(9):861–71.

35. Ayappa I, Norman RG, Rapoport DM. Cardiogenic oscillations on the airflow signal during continuous positive airway pressure as a marker of central apnea. Chest 1999;116(3):660–6.

36. Oostveen E, MacLeod D, Lorino H, et al. The forced oscillation technique in clinical practice: methodology, recommendations and future developments. Eur Respir J 2003;22(6):1026–41.

37. Iber C, Ancoli-Israel S, Chesson AL, et al. The AASM manual for the scoring of sleep and associated events: rules, terminology and technical specications. 1st edition. Westchester (IL): American Academy of Sleep Medicine; 2007.

38. Berry RB, Budhiraja R, Gottlieb DJ, et al. Rules for scoring respiratory events in sleep: update of the 2007 AASM manual for the scoring of sleep and associated events. Deliberations of the sleep apnea definitions task force of the American academy of sleep medicine. J Clin Sleep Med 2012;8(5):597–619.

39. Weiss P, Kryger M. Positive airway pressure therapy for obstructive sleep apnea. Otolaryngol Clin North Am 2016;49(6):1331–41.

40. Battisti A, Tassaux D, Janssens J-P, et al. Performance characteristics of 10 home mechanical ventilators in pressure-support mode: a comparative bench study. Chest 2005;127(5):1784–92.

41. Highcock MP, Shneerson JM, Smith IE. Functional differences in bi-level pressure preset ventilators. Eur Respir J 2001;17(2):268–73.

42. Carteaux G, Lyazidi A, Cordoba-Izquierdo A, et al. Patient-ventilator asynchrony during noninvasive ventilation: a bench and clinical study. Chest 2012;142(2):367–76.

43. Hart DE, Forman M, Veale AG. Effect of tubing condensate on non-invasive positive pressure ventilators tested under simulated clinical conditions. Sleep Breath 2011;15(3):535–41.

44. Rabec C, Georges M, Kabeya NK, et al. Evaluating noninvasive ventilation using a monitoring system coupled to a ventilator: a bench-to-bedside study. Eur Respir J 2009;34(4):902–13.

45. Contal O, Vignaux L, Combescure C, et al. Monitoring of noninvasive ventilation by built-in software of home bilevel ventilators: a bench study. Chest 2012;141(2):469–76.

46. Luján M, Sogo A, Pomares X, et al. Effect of leak and breathing pattern on the accuracy of tidal volume estimation by commercial home ventilators: a bench study. Respir Care 2013;58(5):770–7.

47. Sogo A, Montanyà J, Monsó E, et al. Effect of dynamic random leaks on the monitoring accuracy of home mechanical ventilators: a bench study. BMC Pulm Med 2013;13:75.

48. Olivieri C, Costa R, Conti G, et al. Bench studies evaluating devices for non-invasive ventilation: critical analysis and future perspectives. Intensive Care Med 2011;38(1):160–7.

49. Javaheri S, Brown LK, Randerath WJ. Positive airway pressure therapy with adaptive servoventilation: part 1: operational algorithms. Chest 2014; 146(2):514–23.

50. Meurice JC, Cornette A, Philip-Joet F, et al. Evaluation of autoCPAP devices in home treatment of sleep apnea/hypopnea syndrome. Sleep Med 2007;8(7–8):695–703.

51. Patruno V, Aiolfi S, Costantino G, et al. Fixed and autoadjusting continuous positive airway pressure treatments are not similar in reducing cardiovascular risk factors in patients with obstructive sleep apnea. Chest 2007;131(5):1393–9.

52. Patruno V, Tobaldini E, Bianchi AM, et al. Acute effects of autoadjusting and fixed continuous positive airway pressure treatments on cardiorespiratory coupling in obese patients with obstructive sleep apnea. Eur J Intern Med 2014;25(2):164–8.

53. Karasulu L, Epöztürk PÖ, Sökücü SN, et al. Improving heart rate variability in sleep apnea patients: differences in treatment with auto-titrating positive airway pressure (APAP) versus conventional CPAP. Lung 2010;188(4):315–20.

54. Marrone O, Insalaco G, Bonsignore MR, et al. Sleep structure correlates of continuous positive airway pressure variations during application of an autotitrating continuous positive airway pressure machine in patients with obstructive sleep apnea syndrome. Chest 2002;121(3):759–67.

55. Ip S, D'Ambrosio C, Patel K, et al. Auto-titrating versus fixed continuous positive airway pressure for the treatment of obstructive sleep apnea: a systematic review with meta-analyses. Syst Rev 2012;1:20.

56. Pittman SD, Pillar G, Berry RB, et al. Follow-up assessment of CPAP efficacy in patients with obstructive sleep apnea using an ambulatory device based on peripheral arterial tonometry. Sleep Breath 2006;10(3):123–31.

57. Baltzan MA, Kassissia I, Elkholi O, et al. Prevalence of persistent sleep apnea in patients treated with continuous positive airway pressure. Sleep 2006; 29(4):557–63.

58. Berry RB, Kushida CA, Kryger MH, et al. Respiratory event detection by a positive airway pressure device. Sleep 2012;35(3):361–7.

59. Smith I, Lasserson TJ. Pressure modification for improving usage of continuous positive airway pressure machines in adults with obstructive sleep apnoea. Cochrane Database Syst Rev 2009;(4):CD003531.

60. Aloia MS, Stanchina M, Arnedt JT, et al. Treatment adherence and outcomes in flexible vs standard continuous positive airway pressure therapy. Chest 2005;127(6):2085–93.

61. Nilius G, Happel A, Domanski U, et al. Pressure-relief continuous positive airway pressure vs constant continuous positive airway pressure: a comparison of efficacy and compliance. Chest 2006;130(4): 1018–24.

62. Kakkar RK, Berry RB. Positive airway pressure treatment for obstructive sleep apnea. Chest 2007; 132(3):1057–72.

63. Marshall NS, Neill AM, Campbell AJ. Randomised trial of compliance with flexible (C-Flex) and standard continuous positive airway pressure for severe obstructive sleep apnea. Sleep Breath 2008;12(4): 393–6.

64. Pépin J-L, Muir J-F, Gentina T, et al. Pressure reduction during exhalation in sleep apnea patients treated by continuous positive airway pressure. Chest 2009;136(2):490–7.

65. Brown LK. Achieving adherence to positive airway pressure therapy: modifying pressure and the holy grail. Chest 2011;139(6):1266–8.

66. Bakker JP, Marshall NS. Flexible pressure delivery modification of continuous positive airway pressure for obstructive sleep apnea does not improve compliance with therapy: systematic review and meta-analysis. Chest 2011;139(6):1322–30.

67. Bakker J, Campbell A, Neill A. Randomized controlled trial comparing flexible and continuous positive airway pressure delivery: effects on compliance, objective and subjective sleepiness and vigilance. Sleep 2010;33(4):523–9.

68. Mulgrew AT, Cheema R, Fleetham J, et al. Efficacy and patient satisfaction with autoadjusting CPAP with variable expiratory pressure vs standard CPAP: a two-night randomized crossover trial. Sleep Breath 2006;11(1):31–7.

69. Kushida CA, Berry RB, Blau A, et al. Positive airway pressure initiation: a randomized controlled trial to assess the impact of therapy mode and titration process on efficacy, adherence, and outcomes. Sleep 2011;34(8):1083–92.

70. Chihara Y, Tsuboi T, Hitomi T, et al. Flexible positive airway pressure improves treatment adherence compared with auto-adjusting PAP. Sleep 2013; 36(2):229–36.

71. Cowie MR, Woehrle H, Wegscheider K, et al. Adaptive servo-ventilation for central sleep apnea in systolic heart failure. N Engl J Med 2015;373(12): 1095–105.

72. Leger D, Elbaz M, Piednoir B, et al. Evaluation of the add-on NOWAPI® medical device for remote monitoring of compliance to continuous positive airway pressure and treatment efficacy in obstructive sleep apnea. Biomed Eng Online 2016;15:26.

# Treatment of Obstructive Sleep Apnea

## Choosing the Best Positive Airway Pressure Device

Neil Freedman, MD

### KEYWORDS

- CPAP • Bilevel PAP (BPAP) • AutoPAP (APAP) • AutoBPAP • Expiratory pressure relief
- Humidification • Adherence

### KEY POINTS

- Continuous positive airway pressure (CPAP), autotitrating positive airway pressure (APAP), and bilevel positive airway pressure (BPAP) are all reasonable therapies that can be used for patients with uncomplicated obstructive sleep apnea (OSA) across the spectrum of disease severity.
- All of these therapies can be expected to reduce or resolve sleep-disordered breathing and improve symptoms of daytime sleepiness, with the best outcomes being observed in patients with moderate to severe OSA.
- Unattended APAP, either as chronic treatment or as a method to determine a fixed CPAP setting, should be considered first-line therapy for patients with uncomplicated OSA.
- BPAP should be considered for patients who are nonadherent to CPAP or APAP therapy because of pressure intolerance.
- Other factors that should be considered when choosing a PAP device for a given patient include cost, access to online data management software and patient portals, additional technologies such as heated humidification and expiratory pressure relief, and ease of portability for patients who travel frequently.

## INTRODUCTION

Treatment with positive airway pressure (PAP) remains the primary therapy for most patients with obstructive sleep apnea (OSA), especially those with moderate to severe OSA. This article focuses on how to determine which type of PAP device may be best for treating a given patient or patient population with OSA. Initially, the author reviews the various forms of PAP therapy for the treatment of OSA, including continuous positive airway pressure (CPAP), autotitrating positive airway pressure (APAP), and bilevel positive airway pressure (BPAP) therapies, focusing on their mechanisms of action and indications for use in clinical practice. The remainder of the article focuses on how to determine the best PAP device for a given patient or patient population, evaluating factors such as expected outcomes, ease of use and cost of therapy, application of additional technologies, online data management, patient portals and application-based interfaces and compatibility with other manufacturers interfaces and supplies. This review focuses on types of PAP delivery systems and associated technologies and does

Disclosure Statement: The author has nothing to disclose.
Pulmonary, Critical Care, Allergy and Immunology, Department of Medicine, North Shore University Health System, 2650 Ridge Avenue, Evanston, IL 60201, USA
*E-mail address:* Neilfreedman@comcast.net

Sleep Med Clin 12 (2017) 529–542
http://dx.doi.org/10.1016/j.jsmc.2017.07.003

not make recommendations based on a specific manufacturer because it is not clear from the literature that any one manufacturer's devices are consistently superior. Finally, this article only briefly covers interventions that may improve adherence to therapy and various mask interfaces, because these topics will be covered in depth within their own dedicated articles within this issue.

## TYPES OF POSITIVE AIRWAY PRESSURE DEVICES

Once the clinician has determined that PAP therapy is the best choice for a given patient with OSA, they initially need to decide which type of PAP technology to use, because there are several modes in which PAP therapy can be delivered. These modes include CPAP, APAP, BPAP, and Auto-BPAP.

### Continuous Positive Airway Pressure

CPAP therapy was initially described as a treatment of OSA by Sullivan and colleagues[1] in 1981. Since its initial description, CPAP has become the predominant therapy for the treatment of patients with OSA, because it has been demonstrated to resolve sleep-disordered breathing events and improve several clinical outcomes.[2,3] CPAP delivers a single pressure to the posterior pharynx throughout the night and acts as a pneumatic splint that maintains the patency of the upper airway in a dose-dependent fashion. The best pressure for CPAP treatment is typically determined during an in-laboratory attended sleep study, although a fixed CPAP pressure may also be determined using a short unattended trial of APAP therapy. Treatment with CPAP is typically indicated for patients with moderate to severe OSA (Apnea Hypopnea Index [AHI] $\geq$15 events per hour) with or without associated symptoms or comorbid diseases, and for patients with mild OSA (AHI $\geq$5 to $\leq$14 events per hour) with associated symptoms or comorbid diseases (**Box 1**).

### Autotitrating Positive Airway Pressure

APAP (also known as auto-, automated, auto-adjusting, or automatic) incorporates the ability of the PAP device to detect and respond to changes in upper airway flow or resistance in real time.[4] Currently available APAP devices use proprietary algorithms to noninvasively detect and respond to variations in patterns of upper airway inspiratory flow or resistance. Most APAP machines monitor a combination of changes in inspiratory flow patterns, including inspiratory flow limitation, snoring

---

**Box 1**
**Typical indications for positive airway pressure therapies for obstructive sleep apnea**

- CPAP
  - Moderate to severe OSA ($\geq$15 events per hour of sleep) with or without associated symptoms or comorbid diseases
  - Mild OSA ($\geq$5 to $\leq$14 events per hour of sleep) *with* symptoms or associated comorbid diseases:
    - Symptoms:
      - Excessive daytime sleepiness, impaired cognition, mood disorders or insomnia
    - Comorbid diseases:
      - Hypertension, ischemic heart disease, or history of stroke
- APAP
  - Moderate to severe uncomplicated OSA
  - APAP should *not* be used in patients with complicated OSA
    - Complicated OSA is defined as OSA associated with comorbid medical conditions that could potentially affect their respiratory patterns during sleep, including (1) CHF; (2) Lung diseases such as COPD; and (3) Patients expected to have nocturnal arterial oxyhemoglobin desaturation because of conditions other than OSA (eg, obesity hypoventilation syndrome and other hypoventilation syndromes).
  - May be used in an unattended setting for as the exclusive initial and ongoing therapy
  - May also be used as initial therapy to determine a fixed CPAP setting
- Bilevel PAP
  - May be used for the entire spectrum of OSA severity, although is typically considered for patients who have failed CPAP therapy or have pressure intolerance to other initial PAP therapies
- Auto-bilevel PAP
  - Role in OSA therapy and indications not clear

---

(indirectly measured via mask pressure vibration), reductions of airflow (hypopnea), and absence of flow (apneas), using a pneumotachograph, nasal pressure monitors, or alterations in compressor speed. Another less commonly used technology uses forced oscillation technique (FOT), which is an alternative process that detects changes in patterns of upper airway resistance or impedance.[5–7] Because the FOT method measures changes in upper airway resistance that are independent of patient activity and ventilatory effort, this technology tends to be superior to the flow-based technology at differentiating central apneas from obstructive apneas or mask leak.

Once upper airway flow or impedance changes have been detected, the APAP devices use proprietary algorithms to automatically increase the pressure until the flow or resistance has been normalized. Once a therapeutic pressure has been achieved, the APAP devices typically reduce pressure until flow limitation or increases in airway resistance resume. Most devices have a therapeutic pressure range between 4 cm $H_2O$ and 20 cm $H_2O$, providing the clinician with the ability to adjust the upper and lower pressure limits based on the clinical conditions and the patient's response to therapy. APAP should be differentiated from BPAP or auto-BPAP (discussed later) in which a separate inspiratory positive airway pressure (IPAP) and expiratory positive airway pressure (EPAP) are set with changes in pressure occurring across each respiratory cycle.

Currently available APAP machines have several potential limitations. Most flow/pressure-based APAP devices are somewhat limited in their ability to distinguish between central and obstructive apneas as well as large mask leaks.[8–11] These flow patterns are "interpreted" by these types of devices as an absence of flow, which, in the cases of central apneas and leaks, may erroneously lead to increases in pressure and worsening of the central events or leaks. Newer APAP algorithms appear to be better at differentiating obstructive from central events as well as compensating for large mask leaks. Also the ability of the APAP devices to respond to sustained hypoventilation in the absence of upper airway obstruction is unclear, because most APAP studies have excluded patients at high risk for hypoventilation, including those patients with obesity hypoventilation syndrome or chronic respiratory diseases.[7,12–21] Given these potential limitations in technology as well as the exclusion of patients with many comorbid diseases from the randomized trials comparing APAP to in-laboratory titrated CPAP therapy, APAP devices are typically recommended for patients with uncomplicated moderate to severe OSA.[13,14,22,23] APAP devices can also be used for patients with mild OSA, although there are less data to support the use of APAP in this patient population.[19] APAP devices typically should *not* be used in patients with comorbid medical conditions that could potentially affect their respiratory patterns (complicated OSA) during sleep, including the following: (1) Congestive heart failure (CHF); (2) Lung diseases such as chronic obstructive pulmonary disease (COPD); and (3) patients expected to have nocturnal arterial oxyhemoglobin desaturation due to conditions other than OSA (eg, obesity hypoventilation syndrome and other hypoventilation syndromes). Patients who do not snore (either due to palatal surgery or naturally) should not be titrated with an APAP device that relies on vibration or sound in the device's algorithm.[13,14,22] Finally, APAP devices are not recommended for split-night titrations given the lack of data to support such a practice (see **Box 1**).

## Bilevel Positive Airway Pressure

BPAP therapy's potential benefits in treating patients with OSA were first described in 1990.[24] As opposed to CPAP, which delivers a fixed pressure throughout the respiratory cycle, BPAP therapy allows the independent adjustment of the EPAP and the IPAP. In its initial description, BPAP therapy demonstrated that obstructive events could be eliminated at a lower EPAP compared with conventional CPAP pressures.[24] For patients with uncomplicated OSA, BPAP is typically used in the spontaneous mode (ie, without a back up rate) with an IPAP and EPAP pressure difference of $\geq 4$ cm $H_2O$. To determine the optimal IPAP and EPAP settings, BPAP therapy is typically titrated during an attended in-laboratory sleep study. BPAP may be used for patients with OSA across the spectrum of disease severity, although it is typically recommended as a treatment option for patients with pressure complaints that make it difficult to tolerate CPAP therapy (see **Box 1**). Although intuitively one would predict that BPAP would increase adherence by reducing expiratory pressure–related discomfort and side effects, there are in fact no objective outcomes studies that show that BPAP therapy improves adherence when compared with CPAP therapy for patients with uncomplicated OSA.[25–27] Overall, there have been few studies that objectively evaluate BPAP therapy for the treatment of OSA or compared this mode of PAP therapy to other types of PAP devices for uncomplicated OSA. In addition, there are no short-term or long-term studies evaluating the effects of BPAP on any cardiovascular outcomes in patients with uncomplicated OSA.

## Auto-Bilevel Positive Airway Pressure

Auto-BPAP therapy has also been developed, which, using proprietary algorithms, automatically adjusts both the EPAP and the IPAP in response to sleep-disordered breathing events. Limited data indicate that, compared with CPAP, auto-BPAP therapy results in similar compliance and other important outcomes in patients who have had poor initial experiences with CPAP therapy.[28,29] There is currently no peer-reviewed literature evaluating outcomes with auto-BPAP therapy for OSA in PAP-naive patients. Thus, unlike other modes of PAP therapy, there are no specific indications for auto-BPAP use, and no recommendations can be made for auto-BPAP therapy for treating patients with OSA.

## CHOOSING THE BEST DEVICE BASED ON EXPECTED OUTCOMES

When determining the best PAP device for a given patient with OSA, the clinician should have a reasonable understanding of which outcomes are most important to the patient and which outcomes are most likely to improve based on the patient's symptoms and comorbid medical problems. Although it is the perception of many non–sleep practitioners and the lay public that PAP treatment consistently resolves or improves several important outcomes including sleep architecture, daytime sleepiness, neurocognitive function, mood, quality of life, and cardiovascular disease in all patients with OSA, this is not the case for many patients.

### Resolution of Sleep-Disordered Breathing Events

When titrated appropriately, all types of PAP devices resolve most sleep-disordered breathing across the spectrum of disease severity and have been demonstrated to be superior to placebo, conservative management, and positional therapy with regard to this outcome.[25,26] Randomized controlled trials have also shown CPAP therapy to be superior to placebo at increasing the percent and total time in stages N3 (non–rapid eye movement sleep stage 3) and rapid eye movement (REM) sleep. CPAP's effects on other sleep parameters, including stages N1 and N2 sleep (non–rapid eye movement sleep stages 1 and 2, respectively), total sleep time, and the arousal index, have been inconsistent across studies.[25,26] Compared with standard fixed CPAP therapy, APAP devices as a group are almost always associated with a reduction in mean pressure across a night of therapy in the range of 2 cm $H_2O$ to 2.5 cm $H_2O$, although peak pressures through the night tend to be higher than fixed CPAP therapy. Despite these differences between CPAP and APAP, there are no clinically significant

differences between CPAP and APAP with regards to important outcomes, such as improvements in daytime sleepiness or adherence to therapy.

### Improvement in Daytime Sleepiness

All of the described PAP therapies typically result in significant improvements in subjective symptoms of daytime sleepiness in OSA patients who suffer from this complaint, with the best outcomes being observed in those who suffer from moderate to severe OSA (AHI >15 events per hour).[7,12,15,16,18,19,21,30–51] The minimal and optimal amounts of nocturnal use necessary to improve symptoms of daytime sleepiness are not well defined and appear to be specific to the given individual. Even partial nocturnal use (as little as 2 hours per night) has been associated with significant improvements in daytime symptoms in some patients.[52,53] In general, greater adherence to any of the described PAP therapies on a nightly basis has been associated with greater improvements in symptoms of daytime sleepiness. The data regarding the effects of PAP on more objective measures of daytime sleepiness are more inconsistent across the spectrum of disease severity with results being similar between the different modes of therapy.[21,25,30]

### Improvement in Neurocognitive Function, Mood, and Quality of Life

Numerous studies have assessed the effects of sleep-disordered breathing on neurocognitive functioning, mood, and quality of life.[26,37,54–65] Most randomized controlled studies demonstrate inconsistent improvements in several neurobehavioral performance parameters across the spectrum of disease severity.[25,37,39,54–56,66,67] The data regarding the therapeutic effects of PAP treatment on mood and quality of life are also variable and inconsistent, with many randomized trials demonstrating no clear benefits of CPAP therapy compared with placebo or conservative treatments in these parameters.[25,68] Although it is beyond the scope of this article, there are several potential explanations for the inconsistent improvements in neurocognitive function, mood, and quality of life demonstrated with CPAP therapy.[69]

Despite the inconsistent data regarding improvements in neurocognitive function with PAP use, several observational studies support a significant reduction in the incidence of motor vehicle accidents in symptomatic patients with OSA following the initiation of CPAP therapy.[70,71] Although the actual time course to improved driving performance in real-life situations is not clear, driving simulator performance can improve in as little as 2 to 7 nights of therapy. Similar to other aspects of neurobehavioral performance that may be adversely affected by OSA, many patients with OSA may continue to demonstrate impaired driving simulator performance despite several months of high adherence to CPAP therapy.[72] Unfortunately, there is no specific threshold of CPAP use or duration of treatment that can accurately predict a given individual's fitness to safely drive a vehicle. Because the severity of OSA alone is not a reliable predictor of motor vehicle accident risk, the clinician must take into account several factors including improvements in subjective symptoms and adherence with therapy before determining a driver's ability to safely operate a motor vehicle. Although it is likely that all types of PAP therapies for OSA result in a reduction of motor vehicle accidents, all of the literature on this topic is specific to CPAP therapy.

## Reductions in Hypertension and Cardiovascular Disease

Although untreated OSA has been associated with an increased risk for hypertension and other cardiovascular diseases in certain populations, the literature and outcomes data supporting the beneficial effects of CPAP on cardiovascular outcomes have been inconsistent.[25,26,73–75] Several randomized clinical trials and meta-analyses have assessed the effects of CPAP on blood pressure.[76–79] Overall, CPAP treatment appears to attenuate the adverse effects of untreated OSA on daytime and nocturnal systolic and diastolic blood pressure, and 24-hour mean blood pressure. These data demonstrate that, compared with placebo, sham CPAP, or supportive therapy alone, CPAP treatment is associated with small (−1.8 to −3.0 mm Hg), but statistically significant, improvements in diurnal mean arterial systolic and diastolic blood pressures. In patients with resistant hypertension and OSA, CPAP tends to improve nighttime blood pressure, although the impact of CPAP on daytime blood pressure has been more unpredictable.[80,81] In general, improvements in blood pressure with CPAP therapy have been associated with greater severity of baseline OSA (higher AHI), the presence of subjective daytime sleepiness, younger age, uncontrolled hypertension at baseline, and greater adherence with CPAP use on a nightly basis.

The most convincing long-term data regarding the potential beneficial effects of CPAP therapy on cardiovascular outcomes comes are based on prospective observational data in a large group of male OSA patients with the spectrum of OSA severity and associated daytime sleepiness.[82] Results from this study demonstrated that CPAP treatment (>4 hours per night) in patients with severe OSA (AHI ≥30 events per hour) reduced the incidence of adverse cardiovascular outcomes and improved survival, demonstrating outcomes similar to normal controls. Similar improvements in outcomes with CPAP therapy were not observed in OSA patients with mild to moderate obstructive sleep apnea. Aside from these observational data, there are little data that demonstrate that CPAP therapy as typically used reduces mortality or cardiovascular morbidity and no data that demonstrates that CPAP improves cardiovascular outcomes in patients without associated daytime sleepiness.[75,83]

The role of CPAP therapy in resolving or reducing the occurrence or reoccurrence of cardiac arrhythmias is also uncertain. Several observational studies have demonstrated an association between OSA and atrial fibrillation as well as a higher risk of recurrence of atrial fibrillation after electrical cardioversion or catheter ablation therapy. These studies also have shown an association between increased adherence with CPAP therapy and a lower recurrence rate of atrial fibrillation after these procedures.[84–87] Because all of the current data regarding CPAP therapy and atrial fibrillation are based on observational studies, the role of CPAP as an adjunct treatment to improve atrial arrhythmia control remains uncertain. Although there may be an increased risk of ventricular arrhythmias (tachycardia and fibrillation) in some patients with untreated OSA, there are limited data evaluating the effect of PAP therapy for reducing the incidence and prevalence of these events.[88] Thus, the role of PAP therapy for reducing ventricular arrhythmias in patients with OSA is not clear. As is the case with most of the cardiovascular outcomes literature, the data evaluating the effects of PAP therapy on arrhythmia reduction is specific to CPAP therapy because there are no trials looking at the effects of APAP or BPAP on these outcomes.

Given the inconclusive nature of CPAP therapy on cardiovascular outcomes in general, CPAP therapy should be considered adjunctive therapy to lower blood pressure in hypertensive patients with OSA and daytime symptoms.[26] Several authorities and professional societies have recommended that further supporting data are required to better determine the role of CPAP therapy on improving cardiovascular outcomes before making recommendations for its use in various populations.[73,74] Finally, it should be noted that all of the cardiovascular outcomes data are specific to CPAP therapy. There are no short-term or long-term randomized controlled or prospective observational studies specifically focusing on the impact of APAP, BPAP, or auto-BPAP therapies on any cardiovascular outcomes.

## POSITIVE AIRWAY PRESSURE USE AND OUTCOMES IN SPECIFIC PATIENT POPULATIONS

Most of the outcomes literature related to PAP therapy has focused predominantly on patients with moderate to severe OSA with associated daytime sleepiness and the absence of comorbid medical problems. As all clinicians know, patients with OSA may present with different phenotypes often exhibiting many different symptoms, with or without the presence of one or more comorbid medical conditions.

### Positive Airway Pressure Therapy in Patients with Mild Obstructive Sleep Apnea

As noted previously, most of the literature assessing the effects of PAP on various outcomes has predominantly evaluated OSA patients with moderate to severe disease. Although approximately 28% of patients with mild disease (AHI = 5–14 events per hour) complain of subjective daytime sleepiness,[89] it remains unclear whether treating this group of patients with PAP therapy consistently improves their daytime symptoms. Results from the CPAP Apnea Trial North American Program Trial demonstrated that CPAP therapy significantly improved daytime symptoms as measured by the Functional Outcomes of Sleep Questionnaire (FOSQ) when compared with sham CPAP therapy in symptomatic patients (Mean Epworth Sleepiness Scale score of 15) with mild to moderate OSA over an 8-week period of follow-up.[90] Alternatively, The Apnea Positive Pressure Long Term Efficacy Study showed no significant improvements in objective alertness or subjective sleepiness in patients with mild OSA after 2 and 6 months of CPAP therapy.[39] Limited data evaluating APAP therapy in this patient population have demonstrated some improvement in subjective daytime sleepiness, with results similar to CPAP.[19] Thus, the role of CPAP therapy for this indication in patients with mild disease remains unclear based on the current data.

It appears reasonable to initiate CPAP or APAP therapy in patients with mild OSA and associated daytime sleepiness, but the decision to continue chronic therapy in this patient group should be based on a positive response to therapy. For patients with mild disease without daytime symptoms, it is not clear that treating these patients is beneficial or should be recommended based on the current data.

### The Role of Continuous Positive Airway Pressure Therapy in Patients with Rapid Eye Movement–Predominant Obstructive Sleep Apnea

The prevalence of REM sleep–related or REM-predominant OSA is unclear, in part because of the absence of a standard definition for this entity. This OSA variant tends to be more common in women, although it may affect adult patients of both genders across the age spectrum.[91,92] The association of this OSA variant with daytime or nighttime symptoms is not clear, but it appears that a subgroup of patients is affected. Recent studies have also indicated that REM OSA is independently associated with prevalent and incident hypertension, nondipping of nocturnal blood pressure, increased insulin resistance, and impairment of human spatial navigational memory.[93,94]

For those patients who demonstrate this phenotype of OSA and complain of daytime symptoms or nighttime sleep disturbance, it is unclear if treatment with CPAP consistently improves daytime or nighttime symptoms. Limited observational data of CPAP therapy in symptomatic patients with such REM-predominant OSA have demonstrated significant improvements in daytime sleepiness, fatigue, and functional outcomes as assessed by the FOSQ. These improvements with CPAP therapy were similar to patients with OSA not limited to REM sleep.[91] However, it should be noted, there are no randomized controlled data assessing any outcomes in this subgroup of patients, including cardiovascular disease outcomes, and there are no data evaluating the effects of other types of PAP devices in this patient population.

### Obstructive Sleep Apnea and Comorbid Diseases: Congestive Heart Failure, Chronic Obstructive Pulmonary Disease, Diabetes Mellitus

CHF is a common disease with an estimated prevalence of concomitant OSA of approximately 33%. Several randomized controlled studies have assessed the effects of CPAP therapy on left ventricular ejection fraction (LVEF) in CHF patients with and without systolic dysfunction.[95] Overall, CPAP therapy has shown statistically significant improvements in LVEF in patients with OSA and concomitant systolic dysfunction, with an average improvement in LVEF across studies of approximately 5%. In patients with diastolic CHF and concomitant OSA, CPAP therapy has not been associated with significant improvements in LVEF (1%). However, it is uncertain if the improvements in LVEF in patients with OSA and concomitant CHF translate into improvements in other important outcomes, such as reductions in hospitalizations and mortality. Most of the studies evaluating this patient population have been limited by small sample sizes and relatively short durations of follow-up (typically 12 weeks or less). These findings are limited to CPAP therapy, because APAP is contraindicated in this group of patients, and there are no data evaluating the use of BPAP in this patient population.

The "overlap syndrome" refers to the coexistence of OSA with COPD. Prospective observational data have shown that CPAP therapy in OSA patients with concomitant COPD has been associated with significant reductions in both acute exacerbations of COPD requiring hospitalizations and death with outcomes similar to COPD patients without OSA.[96] Increased adherence to CPAP therapy has been independently associated with reduced mortality in this patient population, whereas decreased CPAP adherence and increased age have been independently associated with increased mortality.[97] Observational data would suggest that adherence to CPAP therapy for as little as 2 hours per night may be associated with a reduction in mortality in this group of patients. Given the current observational data, it is reasonable to recommend CPAP therapy in patients with the overlap syndrome, although given the absence of randomized controlled data in this patient population, the role of CPAP therapy to reduce exacerbations or improve mortality remains undefined. As is the case with CHF, these recommendations are limited to CPAP therapy because APAP therapy is contraindicated in this patient population.

The role of CPAP therapy for improving important outcomes-associated diabetes mellitus (short-term and long-term glucose control) in patients with coexistent OSA is also unclear, because most of the trials evaluating the use of CPAP in this patient population have yielded inconsistent results.[98,99] The role of CPAP as an adjunct therapy to improve weight loss is also uncertain, and adequate treatment of OSA has not been observed to result in enhanced weight loss in most studies.[100] In fact, some studies have demonstrated a small, but significant weight gain with CPAP use, with greater weight gain being associated with increased adherence to CPAP therapy.[101] The role of APAP or BPAP on weight reduction is not clear.

## Positive Airway Pressure in Patients Without Daytime Sleepiness

As noted previously, the presence of subjective daytime sleepiness has generally been associated with a more robust improvement in blood pressure with CPAP therapy. Several large randomized controlled trials have assessed the effect of CPAP therapy in patients with moderate to severe OSA without daytime sleepiness (Epworth Sleepiness Scale score $\leq$10) on various cardiovascular outcomes. In general, CPAP therapy has not been associated with significant improvements in blood pressure, reductions in incident hypertension, or cardiovascular events (nonfatal myocardial infarction or stroke, transient ischemic attack, CHF, or cardiovascular death) or reductions in cardiovascular morbidity or mortality in patients with previously diagnosed cardiovascular diseases.[75,83,102] Thus, the benefit of treating patients with moderate to severe OSA who do not have symptoms of daytime sleepiness with any type of PAP device is unclear and remains to be better defined.

## POSITIVE AIRWAY PRESSURE OUTCOMES SUMMARY

CPAP, APAP, and BPAP treatment consistently improve or resolve OSA events across the spectrum of OSA severity and improve symptoms of daytime sleepiness predominantly in patients with moderate to severe OSA. Improvements in other outcomes are less consistent. Treatment with CPAP has been associated with small reductions in blood pressure, with greater reductions being observed in patients with associated daytime sleepiness, poorly controlled or resistant hypertension, and in those who are more adherent to therapy. The role of any type of PAP therapy for reducing long-term cardiovascular risk or mortality in OSA is uncertain based on the current data. Finally, the role of any type of PAP device for patients without daytime symptoms across the spectrum of OSA severity is undefined.

## ADDITIONAL QUESTIONS TO ADDRESS WHEN CHOOSING A POSITIVE AIRWAY PRESSURE DEVICE

In addition to the type of PAP delivery system and expected outcomes, there are several other issues to consider when choosing a PAP device for a given patient or patient population. Other factors that should be considered include the following: effect of PAP technology on adherence to therapy, additional options to improve comfort, cost of therapy, including the need for an in-laboratory attended polysomnography (PSG), availability of online data management tools and patient interfaces, portability, and compatibility with other manufacturers masks and supplies.

### Effect of Positive Airway Pressure Technology on Adherence to Therapy

Adherence to PAP is typically defined as use $\geq 4$ hours per night on $\geq 70\%$ of the nights.[103] Using this definition, subjective adherence ranges between 65% and 90%, whereas objective measures of PAP adherence have demonstrated use in the range of 40% to 83% with the average nightly use ranging between 4 and 5 hours per night.[104] Unfortunately, there are few if any consistent predictors of short-term or long-term adherence to PAP therapy.

Given the differences in PAP delivery systems and advancements in technology over time, do any of the PAP platforms consistently result in improved adherence to PAP therapy? The short answer to the question is no. Head-to-head studies comparing APAP and BPAP to CPAP have consistently demonstrated similar adherence and improvements in daytime symptoms among the 3 types of PAP delivery modes.[21,105] Thus, the choice of device for a given individual should be based on other factors, such as symptoms, expected outcomes, cost, underlying comorbid medical problems, and other factors that are outlined in this article.

### Additional Options That May Improve Positive Airway Pressure Comfort and Adherence: Heated Humidification and Expiratory Pressure Relief

Given the flow rates generated by most PAP devices, many patients complain of nasal congestion or upper airway dryness without the addition of humidification. Fortunately, most modern-day PAP devices have the capacity to add a humidification system. Although one would assume that heated humidification consistently results in improved adherence with PAP therapy, the data evaluating the effects of heated humidification on adherence to CPAP therapy remain controversial. Although there are some studies that demonstrate that the addition of heated humidification can improve adherence to CPAP therapy, there are several studies demonstrating no improvement in adherence with this intervention.[26,106–110] Patients who tend to benefit the most from the addition of heated humidification are those with symptoms of nasal congestion or rhinitis. Limited data evaluating the role of heated tubing to heated humidification have not consistently shown improvements in adherence in patients with and without nasopharyngeal complaints.[110] With this information in mind, heated humidification should be considered for most patients when initially prescribing a PAP device, given the potential benefits with little associated risks. Patients can determine the level of heated humidification depending on their symptoms and changes in their local environment.

Another common complaint for many patients with OSA who are treated with PAP therapy is the uncomfortable feeling of exhaling against positive pressure. This consequence has been proposed as one conceivable barrier to the long-term acceptance of PAP therapy. Several PAP manufacturers have developed expiratory pressure relief (EPR) systems in an attempt to remedy this potential problem. EPR device technologies allow pressure relief during exhalation with the goal to make PAP therapy more comfortable. EPR technologies briefly reduce the PAP pressure, between 1 cm $H_2O$ and 3 cm $H_2O$, during exhalation before returning the pressure to its set PAP setting before the initiation of inspiration. Certain EPR technologies monitor the patient's airflow during exhalation and reduce the expiratory pressure in response to the airflow and patient effort. The amount of pressure relief varies on a breath-by-breath basis, depending on the actual patient's airflow, and is also dictated by the patient's preference setting on the device.

Although several PAP manufacturers have developed EPR technologies for the market place, only the Philips Respironics (Respironics, Inc, Murrysville, PA, USA) technology (CFLEX) has been extensively evaluated in the peer-reviewed literature.[111–113] Several randomized controlled trials have evaluated the role of CFLEX technology compared with standard CPAP therapy in patients with uncomplicated, predominantly moderate to severe OSA. Overall, the use of such CFLEX technology at fixed pressure relief settings between 1 cm $H_2O$ and 3 cm $H_2O$ has not been associated with improved adherence.[113] In addition, improvements in other commonly measured outcomes (subjective sleepiness, objective alertness, vigilance, or residual OSA) were similar to, but not better than, standard CPAP therapy. Similar results have been observed with a similar technology for APAP devices (AFLEX).[20,114] Despite the lack of convincing outcomes data, most of the current PAP devices have EPR or Flex technologies included as standard additions. Thus, patients should be instructed on how to adjust these technologies and may self-titrate the amount of pressure relief based on comfort.

### Cost of Therapy Including the Need for an In-Laboratory Attended Polysomnography

Current general trends in US health care economics have payers focusing on reducing costs, while improving quality and value. Although the

Affordable Care Act has increased the availability of health insurance, one unfortunate result has been increased out-of-pocket costs for patients in the forms of higher deductibles and increased annual health insurance costs. Finally, as payment systems move away from fee-for-service payment models, management approaches that reduce costs while maintaining or improving quality will become more important. Thus, the clinician needs to be aware of the patient's and health system's (where appropriate) costs, when prescribing PAP therapy for the patient with OSA.

In general, CPAP devices are less expensive than APAP and BPAP devices for patients and payers. The main advantage of APAP therapy is that it can be prescribed and used in an unattended setting obviating the need and costs associated with an in-laboratory titration study. As noted previously, APAP used in the proper patient population results in similar outcomes as CPAP. Thus, when reductions in cost are considered in the management strategy for a given patient or population, APAP should be considered the initial PAP treatment either as a primary therapy or as a method to determine a fixed CPAP setting for ongoing treatment in patients with moderate to severe uncomplicated OSA.[115,116]

### Availability of Online Data Management Tools and Patient Interfaces

Unfortunately, as noted previously, most studies have not been able to identify factors that consistently predict short- or long-term adherence with CPAP therapy.[32,103,117–120] Because adherence with PAP therapy tends to be suboptimal, subjective adherence tends to overestimate objective PAP use, and there are no consistent early predictors of PAP adherence, professional societies currently recommend and many payer policies require, objective adherence data assessment to document adherence with therapy and potentially identify problems that can be addressed.[3] Although most randomized controlled trials have used objective adherence data to monitor outcomes related to PAP therapy, the overall impact of assessing objective compliance data either in person or remotely via a telemedicine approach for all patients on PAP therapy is uncertain.[121,122]

Most of the PAP manufacturers have developed sophisticated online software programs for monitoring several parameters of PAP therapy, including nightly adherence, efficacy of therapy (residual AHI), and problems with mask fit (primarily amount of air leak). Many of the same manufacturers have also developed computer-based patient portals or phone-based applications that allow the patient to monitor their progress with therapy. Despite the absence of outcomes data demonstrating consistent benefits of using this information to improve adherence to therapy, the author's group finds this information invaluable for managing patients on a day-to-day basis. Factors to consider when choosing a specific manufacturer's software should include ease of use for the clinician and the patient, compatibility with a given electronic medical record system, and the ability to monitor progress and make adjustments remotely. In reality, most clinicians will need to get comfortable using more than one data-management system given the array of PAP manufacturers currently on the market.

### Portability and Compatibility with Other Manufacturers Masks and Supplies

Practical issues to consider when prescribing a PAP device include the patient's occupation and travel plans as it relates to the ease of portability. Most modern-day PAP devices, regardless of delivery technology, are approximately similar in size and weight when considering the PAP device and supplies. More recently, several companies market much smaller CPAP and APAP devices that may be more suitable for patients who frequently travel for their job or leisure. It is not clear if these smaller portable PAP devices will be durable enough for everyday use. Finally, because it is common for patients to use masks made by different manufacturers, it is good to know that most current PAP devices are compatible with masks made by several manufacturers.

### SUMMARY

CPAP, APAP, and BPAP all are reasonable therapies that can be used for patients with uncomplicated OSA across the spectrum of disease severity. All of these therapies can be expected to reduce or resolve sleep-disordered breathing and improve symptoms of daytime sleepiness, with the best outcomes to be expected in patients with moderate to severe OSA. Unattended APAP, either as chronic treatment or as a method to determine a fixed CPAP setting, should be considered first-line therapy for patients with uncomplicated OSA when the cost of treatment is a priority for the patient. BPAP should be considered for patients who are nonadherent to CPAP or APAP therapy because of pressure intolerance. When choosing the best PAP device for a given patient, the clinician should consider several other factors including cost of the device and management strategy, access to online data management software and patient portals, additional technologies such as heated humidification and EPR, ease of portability for patients who travel frequently, and compatibility with other manufacturers' supplies.

## REFERENCES

1. Sullivan C, Issa F, Berthon-Jones M, et al. Reversal of obstructive sleep apnea by continuous positive airway pressure applied through the nares. Lancet 1981;1:862–5.
2. Loube DI, Gay PC, Strohl KP, et al. Indications for positive airway pressure treatment of adult obstructive sleep apnea patients: a consensus statement. Chest 1999;115(3):863–6.
3. Epstein LJ, Kristo D, Strollo PJ Jr, et al. Clinical guideline for the evaluation, management and long-term care of obstructive sleep apnea in adults. J Clin Sleep Med 2009;5(3):263–76.
4. Roux F, Hilbert J. Continuous positive airway pressure: new generations. In: Lee-Chiong T, Mohsenin V, editors. Clinics in chest medicine, vol. 24. Philadelphia: W.B. Saunders Company; 2003. p. 315–42.
5. Randerath WJ, Parys K, Feldmeyer F, et al. Self-adjusting nasal continuous positive airway pressure therapy based on measurement of impedance: a comparison of two different maximum pressure levels. Chest 1999;116(4):991–9.
6. Randerath WJ, Schraeder O, Galetke W, et al. Autoadjusting CPAP therapy based on impedance efficacy, compliance and acceptance. Am J Respir Crit Care Med 2001;163(3):652–7.
7. Randerath W, Galetke W, David M, et al. Prospective randomized comparison of impedance-controlled auto-continuous positive airway pressure (APAP(FOT)) with constant CPAP. Sleep Med 2001;2:115–24.
8. Abdenbi F, Chambille B, Escourrou P. Bench testing of auto-adjusting positive airway pressure devices. Eur Respir J 2004;24(4):649–58.
9. Rigau J, Montserrat JM, Wohrle H, et al. Bench model to simulate upper airway obstruction for analyzing automatic continuous positive airway pressure devices. Chest 2006;130(2):350–61.
10. Farre R, Montserrat JM, Rigau J, et al. Response of automatic continuous positive airway pressure devices to different sleep breathing patterns: a bench study. Am J Respir Crit Care Med 2002;166(4):469–73.
11. Lofaso F, Desmarais G, Leroux K, et al. Bench evaluation of flow limitation detection by automated continuous positive airway pressure devices. Chest 2006;130(2):343–9.
12. Hudgel DW, Fung C. A long-term randomized cross-over comparison of auto-titrating and standard nasal continuous positive airway pressure. Sleep 2000;23:1–4.
13. Berry R, Parish J, Hartse K. The use of auto-titrating continuous positive airway pressure for the treatment of adult obstructive sleep apnea. Sleep 2002;25(2):148–73.
14. Littner M, Hirshkowitz M, Davilla D, et al. Practice parameters for the use of autotitrating continuous positive airway pressure devices for titrating pressures and treating adult patients with obstructive sleep apnea syndrome. Sleep 2002;25(2):143–7.
15. Ayas N, Patel S, Malhotra A, et al. Auto-titrating vs standard continuous positive airway pressure for the treatment of obstructive sleep apnea: results of a meta-analysis. Sleep 2004;27(2):249–53.
16. Hukins CA. Comparative study of autotitrating and fixed-pressure CPAP in the home: a randomized, single-blind crossover trial. Sleep 2004;27(8):1512–7.
17. Stammnitz A, Jerrentrup A, Penzel T, et al. Automatic CPAP titration with different self-setting devices in patients with obstructive sleep apnoea. Eur Respir J 2004;24(2):273–8.
18. Nussbaumer Y, Bloch KE, Genser T, et al. Equivalence of autoadjusted and constant continuous positive airway pressure in home treatment of sleep apnea. Chest 2006;129(3):638–43.
19. Nolan G, Doherty L, McNicholas W. Auto-adjusting versus fixed positive pressure therapy in mild to moderate obstructive sleep apnoea. Sleep 2007;30(2):189–94.
20. Kushida CA, Berry RB, Blau A, et al. Positive airway pressure initiation: a randomized controlled trial to assess the impact of therapy mode and titration process on efficacy, adherence, and outcomes. Sleep 2011;34(8):1083–92.
21. Ip S, D'Ambrosio C, Patel K, et al. Auto-titrating versus fixed continuous positive airway pressure for the treatment of obstructive sleep apnea: a systematic review with meta-analyses. Syst Rev 2012;1:20.
22. Morgenthaler T, Aurora R, Brown T, et al. Practice parameters for the use of autotitrating continuous positive airway pressure devices for titrating pressures and treating adult patients with obstructive sleep apnea syndrome: an update for 2007. An American Academy of Sleep Medicine report. Sleep 2008;31:141–7.
23. Freedman N. Positive airway pressure therapy for obstructive sleep apnea. In: Kyrger MRT, Dement W, editors. The principles and practice of sleep medicine. 6th edition. New York: Elsevier Saunders Press; 2016. p. 1125–37.
24. Sanders M, Kern N. Obstructive sleep apnea treated by independently adjusted inspiratory and expiratory positive airway pressures via nasal mask. Physiologic and clinical implications. Chest 1990;98(2):317–24.
25. Gay P, Weaver T, Loube D, et al. Evaluation of positive airway pressure treatment for sleep related

breathing disorders in adults. Sleep 2006;29(3): 381–401.

26. Kushida C, Littner M, Hirshkowitz M, et al. Practice parameters for the use of continuous and bilevel positive airway pressure devices to treat adult patients with sleep-related breathing disorders. Sleep 2006;29(3):375–80.

27. Reeves-Hoche M, Hudgel D, Meck R, et al. Continuous versus bilevel positive airway pressure for obstructive sleep apnea. Am J Respir Crit Care Med 1995;151(2):443–9.

28. Carlucci A, Ceriana P, Mancini M, et al. Efficacy of bilevel-auto treatment in patients with obstructive sleep apnea not responsive to or intolerant of continuous positive airway pressure ventilation. J Clin Sleep Med 2015;11(9):981–5.

29. Powell ED, Gay PC, Ojile JM, et al. A pilot study assessing adherence to auto-bilevel following a poor initial encounter with CPAP. J Clin Sleep Med 2012;8(1):43–7.

30. Patel SR, White DP, Malhotra A, et al. Continuous positive airway pressure therapy for treating sleepiness in a diverse population with obstructive sleep apnea: results of a meta-analysis. Arch Intern Med 2003;163(5):565–71.

31. Engleman HM, Douglas NJ. Sleep 4: sleepiness, cognitive function, and quality of life in obstructive sleep apnoea/hypopnoea syndrome. Thorax 2004; 59(7):618–22.

32. Douglas NJ, Engleman HM. CPAP therapy: outcomes and patient use. Thorax 1998;53(90003): 47S–8S.

33. Douglas NJ. Systematic review of the efficacy of nasal CPAP. Thorax 1998;53(5):414–5.

34. Jenkinson C, Davies R, Mullins R, et al. Comparison of therapeutic and subtherapeutic nasal continuous airway pressure for obstructive sleep apnea: a randomized prospective parallel trial. Lancet 1999;353:2100–5.

35. Ballester E, Badia JR, Hernandez L, et al. Evidence of the effectiveness of continuous positive airway pressure in the treatment of sleep apnea/hypopnea syndrome. Am J Respir Crit Care Med 1999;159(2): 495–501.

36. Masa JF, Jimenez A, Duran J, et al. Alternative methods of titrating continuous positive airway pressure: a large multicenter study. Am J Respir Crit Care Med 2004;170(11):1218–24.

37. Engleman H, Martin S, Kingshott R, et al. Randomised, placebo-controlled trial of daytime function after continuous positive airway pressure therapy for the sleep apnoea/hypopnoea syndrome. Thorax 1998;53:341–5.

38. Berry R, Hill G, Thompson L, et al. Portable monitoring and autotitration versus polysomnography for the diagnosis and treatment of sleep apnea. Sleep 2008;31(10):1423–31.

39. Kushida CA, Nichols DA, Holmes TH, et al. Effects of continuous positive airway pressure on neurocognitive function in obstructive sleep apnea patients: the apnea positive pressure long-term efficacy study (APPLES). Sleep 2012;35(12): 1593–602.

40. Schwartz SW, Rosas J, Iannacone MR, et al. Correlates of a prescription for bilevel positive airway pressure for treatment of obstructive sleep apnea among veterans. J Clin Sleep Med 2013;9(4): 327–35.

41. Massie CA, McArdle N, Hart RW, et al. Comparison between automatic and fixed positive airway pressure therapy in the home. Am J Respir Crit Care Med 2003;167(1):20–3.

42. Teschler H, Wessendorf T, Farhat A, et al. Two months auto-adjusting versus conventional nCPAP for obstructive sleep apnoea syndrome. Eur Respir J 2000;15(6):990–5.

43. Meurice J, Marc I, Series F. Efficacy of auto-CPAP in the treatment of obstructive sleep apnea/hypopnea syndrome. Am J Respir Crit Care Med 1996;153(2):794–8.

44. Series F, Marc I. Efficacy of automatic continuous positive airway pressure therapy that uses an estimated required pressure in the treatment of the obstructive sleep apnea syndrome. Ann Intern Med 1997;127(8 Pt 1):588–95.

45. d'Ortho M-P, Grillier-Lanoir V, Levy P, et al. Constant vs automatic continuous positive airway pressure therapy: home evaluation. Chest 2000;118(4): 1010–7.

46. Konermann M, Sanner B, Vyleta M, et al. Use of conventional and self-adjusting nasal continuous positive airway pressure for treatment of severe obstructive sleep apnea syndrome: a comparative study. Chest 1998;113(3):714–8.

47. Planes C, d'Ortho M, Foucher A, et al. Efficacy and cost of home-initiated auto-nCPAP versus conventional nCPAP. Sleep 2003;26(2):156–60.

48. Noseda A, Kempenaers C, Kerkhofs M, et al. Constant vs auto-continuous positive airway pressure in patients with sleep apnea hypopnea syndrome and a high variability in pressure requirement. Chest 2004;126(1):31–7.

49. Pevernagie DA, Proot PM, Hertegonne KB, et al. Efficacy of flow- vs impedance-guided autoadjustable continuous positive airway pressure: a randomized cross-over trial. Chest 2004;126(1): 25–30.

50. Smith I, Lasserson T. Pressure modification for improving usage of systematic age of continuous positive airway pressure machines in adults with obstructive sleep apnoea. Cochrane Database Rev 2009;(4):CD003531.

51. Vennelle M, White S, Riha RL, et al. Randomized controlled trial of variable-pressure versus fixed-

pressure continuous positive airway pressure (CPAP) treatment for patients with obstructive sleep apnea/hypopnea syndrome (OSAHS). Sleep 2010;33(2):267–71.

52. Weaver T, Maislin G, Dinges D, et al. Relationship between hours of CPAP use and achieving normal levels of sleepiness and daily functioning. Sleep 2007;30:711–9.

53. Antic NA, Catcheside P, Buchan C, et al. The effect of CPAP in normalizing daytime sleepiness, quality of life, and neurocognitive function in patients with moderate to severe OSA. Sleep 2011;34(1):111–9.

54. Engleman H, Martin S, Deary I, et al. The effect of continuous positive airway pressure therapy on daytime function in the sleep apnoea/hyponoea syndrome. Lancet 1994;343:572–5.

55. Engleman H, Martin S, Deary I, et al. Effect of CPAP therapy on daytime function in patients with mild sleep apnoea/hypopnoea syndrome. Thorax 1997;52:114–9.

56. Engleman H, Kingshott R, Wraith P, et al. Randomized placebo-controlled crossover trial of CPAP for mild sleep apnea/hypopnea syndrome. Am J Respir Crit Care Med 1999;159:461–7.

57. Engleman H, Kingshott R, Martin S, et al. Cognitive function in the sleep apnea/hyponea syndrome (SAHS). Sleep 2000;23(Suppl 4):S102–8.

58. Greenberg G, Watson R, Deptula D. Neuropsychological dysfunction in sleep apnea. Sleep 1987;10:254–62.

59. Redline S, Strauss M, Adams N, et al. Neuropsychological function in mild sleep-disordered breathing. Sleep 1997;20:160–7.

60. Kim H, Young T, Matthews C, et al. Sleep-disordered breathing and neuropsychological deficits: a population based study. Am J Respir Crit Care Med 1997;156:1813–9.

61. Bedard M, Montplaisir J, Richer F, et al. Obstructive sleep apnea syndrome: pathogenesis of neuropsychological deficits. J Clin Exp Neuropsychol 1991;13:950–64.

62. Borak J, Cieslicki J, Koziej M, et al. Effects of CPAP treatment on psychological status in patients with severe obstructive sleep apnea. J Sleep Res 1996;5(2):123–7.

63. Naegele B, Thouvard V, Pepin J, et al. Deficits of cognitive executive functions in patients with sleep apnea syndrome. Sleep 1995;18:43–52.

64. Ramos Platon M, Espinar Sierra J. Changes in psychopathological symptoms in sleep apnea patients after treatment with nasal continuous airway pressure. Int J Neurosci 1992;62(3–4):173–95.

65. Munoz A, Mayoralas L, Barbe F, et al. Long-term effects of CPAP on daytime functioning in patients with sleep apnoea syndrome. Eur Respir J 2000;15(4):676–81.

66. Zimmerman ME, Arnedt JT, Stanchina M, et al. Normalization of memory performance and positive airway pressure adherence in memory-impaired patients with obstructive sleep apnea. Chest 2006;130(6):1772–8.

67. Olaithe M, Bucks RS. Executive dysfunction in OSA before and after treatment: a meta-analysis. Sleep 2013;36(9):1297–305.

68. Batool-Anwar S, Goodwin JL, Kushida CA, et al. Impact of continuous positive airway pressure (CPAP) on quality of life in patients with obstructive sleep apnea (OSA). J Sleep Res 2016;25(6):731–8.

69. Quan SF, Chan CS, Dement WC, et al. The association between obstructive sleep apnea and neurocognitive performance–the Apnea Positive Pressure Long-term Efficacy Study (APPLES). Sleep 2011;34(3):303–314b.

70. Tregear S, Reston J, Schoelles K, et al. Continuous positive airway pressure reduces risk of motor vehicle crash among drivers with obstructive sleep apnea: systematic review and meta-analysis. Sleep 2010;33(10):1373–80.

71. Ayas N, Skomro R, Blackman A, et al. Obstructive sleep apnea and driving: a Canadian Thoracic Society and Canadian Sleep Society position paper. Can Respir J 2014;21(2):114–23.

72. Vakulin A, Baulk SD, Catcheside PG, et al. Driving simulator performance remains impaired in patients with severe OSA after CPAP treatment. J Clin Sleep Med 2011;7(3):246–53.

73. Gottlieb DJ, Craig SE, Lorenzi-Filho G, et al. Sleep apnea cardiovascular clinical trials-current status and steps forward: the International collaboration of sleep apnea cardiovascular trialists. Sleep 2013;36(7):975–80.

74. Parati G, Lombardi C, Hedner J, et al. Position paper on the management of patients with obstructive sleep apnea and hypertension: joint recommendations by the European Society of Hypertension, by the European Respiratory Society and by the members of European COST (COoperation in Scientific and Technological research) ACTION B26 on obstructive sleep apnea. J Hypertens 2012;30(4):633–46.

75. McEvoy RD, Antic NA, Heeley E, et al. CPAP for prevention of cardiovascular events in obstructive sleep apnea. N Engl J Med 2016;375(10):919–31.

76. Fava C, Dorigoni S, Dalle Vedove F, et al. Effect of CPAP on blood pressure in patients with OSA/hypopnea a systematic review and meta-analysis. Chest 2014;145(4):762–71.

77. Montesi SB, Edwards BA, Malhotra A, et al. The effect of continuous positive airway pressure treatment on blood pressure: a systematic review and meta-analysis of randomized controlled trials. J Clin Sleep Med 2012;8(5):587–96.

78. Haentjens P, Van Meerhaeghe A, Moscariello A, et al. The impact of continuous positive airway pressure on blood pressure in patients with obstructive sleep apnea syndrome: evidence from a meta-analysis of placebo-controlled randomized trials. Arch Intern Med 2007;167(8):757–64.

79. Bakker JP, Edwards BA, Gautam SP, et al. Blood pressure improvement with continuous positive airway pressure is independent of obstructive sleep apnea severity. J Clin Sleep Med 2014; 10(4):365–9.

80. Pepin JL, Tamisier R, Barone-Rochette G, et al. Comparison of continuous positive airway pressure and valsartan in hypertensive patients with sleep apnea. Am J Respir Crit Care Med 2010;182(7): 954–60.

81. Muxfeldt ES, Margallo V, Costa LM, et al. Effects of continuous positive airway pressure treatment on clinic and ambulatory blood pressures in patients with obstructive sleep apnea and resistant hypertension: a randomized controlled trial. Hypertension 2015;65(4):736–42.

82. Marin J, Carrizo S, Vincente E, et al. Long-term cardiovascular outcomes in men with obstructive sleep apnoea-hypopnea with or without treatment with continuous positive airway pressure: an observational study. Lancet 2005;365(9464):1046–53.

83. Barbe F, Duran-Cantolla J, Sanchez-de-la-Torre M, et al. Effect of continuous positive airway pressure on the incidence of hypertension and cardiovascular events in nonsleepy patients with obstructive sleep apnea: a randomized controlled trial. JAMA 2012;307(20):2161–8.

84. Holmqvist F, Guan N, Zhu Z, et al. Impact of obstructive sleep apnea and continuous positive airway pressure therapy on outcomes in patients with atrial fibrillation-results from the outcomes registry for better informed treatment of atrial fibrillation (ORBIT-AF). Am Heart J 2015;169(5):647–54.e2.

85. Fein AS, Shvilkin A, Shah D, et al. Treatment of obstructive sleep apnea reduces the risk of atrial fibrillation recurrence after catheter ablation. J Am Coll Cardiol 2013;62(4):300–5.

86. Kanagala R, Murali NS, Friedman PA, et al. Obstructive sleep apnea and the recurrence of atrial fibrillation. Circulation 2003;107(20):2589–94.

87. Ng CY, Liu T, Shehata M, et al. Meta-analysis of obstructive sleep apnea as predictor of atrial fibrillation recurrence after catheter ablation. Am J Cardiol 2011;108(1):47–51.

88. Raghuram A, Clay R, Kumbam A, et al. A systematic review of the association between obstructive sleep apnea and ventricular arrhythmias. J Clin Sleep Med 2014;10(10):1155–60.

89. Kapur VK, Baldwin CM, Resnick HE, et al. Sleepiness in patients with moderate to severe sleep-disordered breathing. Sleep 2005;28(4):472–7.

90. Weaver TE, Mancini C, Maislin G, et al. Continuous positive airway pressure treatment of sleepy patients with milder obstructive sleep apnea: results of the CPAP Apnea Trial North American Program (CATNAP) randomized clinical trial. Am J Respir Crit Care Med 2012;186(7):677–83.

91. Su CS, Liu KT, Panjapornpon K, et al. Functional outcomes in patients with REM-related obstructive sleep apnea treated with positive airway pressure therapy. J Clin Sleep Med 2012;8(3):243–7.

92. Khan A, Harrison SL, Kezirian EJ, et al. Obstructive sleep apnea during rapid eye movement sleep, daytime sleepiness, and quality of life in older men in Osteoporotic Fractures in Men (MrOS) Sleep Study. J Clin Sleep Med 2013; 9(3):191–8.

93. Mokhlesi B, Hagen EW, Finn LA, et al. Obstructive sleep apnoea during REM sleep and incident non-dipping of nocturnal blood pressure: a longitudinal analysis of the Wisconsin sleep cohort. Thorax 2015;70(11):1062–9.

94. Alzoubaidi M, Mokhlesi B. Obstructive sleep apnea during rapid eye movement sleep: clinical relevance and therapeutic implications. Curr Opin Pulm Med 2016;22(6):545–54.

95. Sun H, Shi J, Li M, et al. Impact of continuous positive airway pressure treatment on left ventricular ejection fraction in patients with obstructive sleep apnea: a meta-analysis of randomized controlled trials. PLoS One 2013;8(5):e62298.

96. Marin JM, Soriano JB, Carrizo SJ, et al. Outcomes in patients with chronic obstructive pulmonary disease and obstructive sleep apnea: the overlap syndrome. Am J Respir Crit Care Med 2010;182(3): 325–31.

97. Stanchina ML, Welicky LM, Donat W, et al. Impact of CPAP use and age on mortality in patients with combined COPD and obstructive sleep apnea: the overlap syndrome. J Clin Sleep Med 2013; 9(8):767–72.

98. Iftikhar IH, Hoyos CM, Phillips CL, et al. Meta-analyses of the association of sleep apnea with insulin resistance, and the effects of CPAP on HOMA-IR, adiponectin, and visceral adipose fat. J Clin Sleep Med 2015;11(4):475–85.

99. Pamidi S, Wroblewski K, Stepien M, et al. Eight hours of nightly CPAP treatment of obstructive sleep apnea improves glucose metabolism in prediabetes: a randomized controlled trial. Am J Respir Crit Care Med 2015;192(1):96–105.

100. Redenius R, Murphy C, O'Neill E, et al. Does CPAP lead to change in BMI? J Clin Sleep Med 2008;4(3): 205–9.

101. Quan SF, Budhiraja R, Clarke DP, et al. Impact of treatment with continuous positive airway pressure (CPAP) on weight in obstructive sleep apnea. J Clin Sleep Med 2013;9(10):989–93.

102. Martinez-Garcia MA, Capote F, Campos-Rodriguez F, et al. Effect of CPAP on blood pressure in patients with obstructive sleep apnea and resistant hypertension: the HIPARCO randomized clinical trial. JAMA 2013;310(22):2407–15.

103. Kribbs N, Pack A, Kline L, et al. Objective measurement of patterns of nasal CPAP use by patients with obstructive sleep apnea. Am Rev Respir Dis 1993; 147:887–95.

104. Parthasarathy S, Subramanian S, Quan SF. A multicenter prospective comparative effectiveness study of the effect of physician certification and center accreditation on patient-centered outcomes in obstructive sleep apnea. J Clin Sleep Med 2014;10(3):243–9.

105. Mansukhani MP, Kolla BP, Olson EJ, et al. Bilevel positive airway pressure for obstructive sleep apnea. Expert Rev Med Devices 2014;11(3):283–94.

106. Massie CA, Hart RW, Peralez K, et al. Effects of humidification on nasal symptoms and compliance in sleep apnea patients using continuous positive airway pressure. Chest 1999;116(2):403–8.

107. Martins de Araujo MT, Vieira SB, Vasquez EC, et al. Heated humidification or face mask to prevent upper airway dryness during continuous positive airway pressure therapy. Chest 2000;117(1):142–7.

108. Rakotonanahary D, Pelletier-Fleury N, Gagnadoux F, et al. Predictive factors for the need for additional humidification during nasal continuous positive airway pressure therapy. Chest 2001;119(2):460–5.

109. Ryan S, Doherty LS, Nolan GM, et al. Effects of heated humidification and topical steroids on compliance, nasal symptoms, and quality of life in patients with obstructive sleep apnea syndrome using nasal continuous positive airway pressure. J Clin Sleep Med 2009;5(5):422–7.

110. Nilius G, Franke KJ, Domanski U, et al. Effect of APAP and heated humidification with a heated breathing tube on adherence, quality of life, and nasopharyngeal complaints. Sleep Breath 2016; 20(1):43–9.

111. Aloia MS, Stanchina M, Arnedt JT, et al. Treatment adherence and outcomes in flexible vs standard continuous positive airway pressure therapy. Chest 2005;127(6):2085–93.

112. Nilius G, Happel A, Domanski U, et al. Pressure-relief continuous positive airway pressure vs constant continuous positive airway pressure: a comparison of efficacy and compliance. Chest 2006;130(4):1018–24.

113. Bakker JP, Marshall NS. Flexible pressure delivery modification of continuous positive airway pressure for obstructive sleep apnea does not improve compliance with therapy: systematic review and meta-analysis. Chest 2011;139(6):1322–30.

114. Dungan GC 2nd, Marshall NS, Hoyos CM, et al. A randomized crossover trial of the effect of a novel method of pressure control (SensAwake) in automatic continuous positive airway pressure therapy to treat sleep disordered breathing. J Clin Sleep Med 2011;7(3):261–7.

115. Parish JM, Freedman NS, Manaker S. Evolution in reimbursement for sleep studies and sleep centers. Chest 2015;147(3):600–6.

116. Freedman N. COUNTERPOINT: does laboratory polysomnography yield better outcomes than home sleep testing? No. Chest 2015;148(2):308–10.

117. Reeves-Hoche M, Meck R, Zwillich C. Nasal CPAP: an objective evaluation of patient compliance. Am J Respir Crit Care Med 1994;149(1):149–54.

118. Rauscher H, Formanek D, Popp W, et al. Self-reported vs measured compliance with nasal CPAP for obstructive sleep apnea. Chest 1993;103(6):1675–80.

119. Engleman H, Martin S, Douglas N. Compliance with CPAP therapy in patients with the sleep apnoea/hypopnoea syndrome. Thorax 1994;49(3):263–6.

120. Rosen CL, Auckley D, Benca R, et al. A multisite randomized trial of portable sleep studies and positive airway pressure autotitration versus laboratory-based polysomnography for the diagnosis and treatment of obstructive sleep apnea: the HomePAP study. Sleep 2012;35(6):757–67.

121. Sparrow D, Aloia M, Demolles DA, et al. A telemedicine intervention to improve adherence to continuous positive airway pressure: a randomised controlled trial. Thorax 2010;65(12):1061–6.

122. Fox N, Hirsch-Allen AJ, Goodfellow E, et al. The impact of a telemedicine monitoring system on positive airway pressure adherence in patients with obstructive sleep apnea: a randomized controlled trial. Sleep 2012;35(4):477–81.

# Treatment of Obstructive Sleep Apnea
## Choosing the Best Interface

Marie Nguyen Dibra, MD[a],*, Richard Barnett Berry, MD[b],
Mary H. Wagner, MD[c]

## KEYWORDS

- OSA • CPAP interface • Nasal mask • Mask fitting • PAP initiation • PAP compliance • Mask leak

## KEY POINTS

- Difficulty with the mask interface is common and no one type of mask is clearly superior. Changing mask type or improving fit to can dramatically improve adherence and satisfaction.
- Trying several mask types and sizes may improve mask seal and comfort; fitting a mask under pressure is suggested (ideally with the patient reclining).
- An oronasal mask may be useful in patients with mouth leak or severe nasal congestion; however, a higher pressure may be needed when switching from a nasal mask to an oronasal mask.
- Hybrid masks may be helpful in patients who could benefit from an oronasal mask but in whom claustrophobia or obtaining a good seal around the upper nose is difficult.
- Proper adjustment, cleaning, and replacement are important for maintaining a good seal. When a mask worked initially but begins to leak over time, the cushion may have deteriorated.

## OVERVIEW

There is a range of interface or mask options available for delivering positive pressure therapy in obstructive sleep apnea (OSA). These include masks that fit into the nostrils (nasal pillows) or that cover the nose (nasal mask), are inserted into the mouth, cover both the nose and the mouth (oronasal mask or full face mask), or even the entire face (total face mask or helmet).[1–3] Adherence to continuous positive airway pressure (CPAP) is a crucial aspect of therapy and the benefits of positive airway pressure (PAP) are most evident in patients who comply with treatment and have longer durations of CPAP use.

Nevertheless, an estimated 46% to 83% of patients are nonadherent with CPAP when compliance is defined as usage for 4 or more hours a night.[2] Predictors of adherence to CPAP therapy include the severity of OSA, the degree of daytime sleepiness, the socioeconomic status, the level of patient understanding of the therapy, and the type of mask used.[3]

It can be challenging to find a mask that fits well and is, at the same time, comfortable to wear. Patients receiving nasal CPAP often complain about side effects related to mask fit such as eye irritation owing to air leak into the eyes, skin reactions to the cushion material, pain or abrasion to the

Disclosures: The authors listed above have identified no professional or financial affiliations for themselves or their spouse/partner.
[a] Division of Pulmonary, Critical Care, and Sleep Medicine, Department of Sleep Medicine, UF Health Sleep Center, University of Florida, 4740 Northwest 39th Place, Gainesville, FL 32606, USA; [b] Department of Sleep Medicine, UF Health Sleep Center, University of Florida, 4740 Northwest 39th Place, Gainesville, FL 32606, USA; [c] Department of Sleep Medicine, UF Health Sleep Disorders Center, UF Health Sleep Center, 4740 Northwest 39th Place, Gainesville, FL 32606, USA
* Corresponding author.
*E-mail address:* Marie.Nguyen@medicine.ufl.edu

Sleep Med Clin 12 (2017) 543–549
http://dx.doi.org/10.1016/j.jsmc.2017.07.004

bridge of the nose, residual imprints on the face in the morning owing to pressure from mask or straps, or pressure sores and noisy air leaks, all of which reduce the tolerability of treatment. A change in mask type or size may be a required to intervene for these problems. Changes in interface may also be needed if the patient develops chronic skin irritation at the point of contact with the mask, if changes in the patient's weight that compromise the mask's fit, or if increases in pressure lead to increased leak issues.[1] For patients who experience symptomatic mouth leak while wearing a nasal mask, the addition of a chin strap or change to an oral nasal interface may be helpful.

## MASK TYPE

A nasal mask is usually the first interface tried for PAP titration and treatment (**Fig. 1**). The biggest challenge with a nasal mask is providing a comfortable seal around the nasal bridge. Given the large variability in the shape and size of noses and the associated nasal bridge, it is not surprising that several masks must often be tried before a satisfactory seal can be obtained. Air leak into the eyes is poorly tolerated by patients. For a nasal mask to work well, the patient must be able to breathe nasally with the mouth closed. If more than a mild degree of expiratory venting through the mouth occurs during sleep, this may result in dryness or arouse the patient frequently. Oronasal masks are an alternative interface that can be used for patients with significant nasal congestion and predominant oral breathing or those with a large mouth leak during sleep.[4] However, an oronasal interface must seal over a large area, which can make finding a good fit very difficult in some patients. In edentulous patients, there is a lack of structural support under the lower face for oronasal masks. In these patients, oronasal masks may compress soft tissues and create an air leak. Several studies have found that oronasal masks generally require a higher treatment pressure than nasal masks and are associated with higher leak or a higher residual apnea–hypopnea index. In an occasional patient, a substantially lower pressure may be effective with a nasal mask compared with a full face mask.[5] It has been hypothesized that use of an oronasal mask may cause the jaw or tongue to move posteriorly, narrowing the upper airway. In addition, some patients may not tolerate an oronasal mask owing to claustrophobia or difficulty obtaining a mask seal. Hybrid masks, which use nasal pillows or a nasal cradle combined with a portion of the mask covering the mouth may be a solution in some patients. Only the lower part of the nose fits down into the cradle, the bottom of which contains an opening hole, allowing air to enter and leave the nares. This type of mask also avoids the need to maintain a seal in the nasal bridge area. For example, the Amara View (Philips Respironics, Murrysville, PA; **Fig. 2**) uses a nasal cradle cushion on top of a portion of the mask that covers the mouth.

Nasal pillows consist of 2 nasal inserts and have emerged as an alternative to nasal masks because they are smaller and have less contact with the face.[3] CPAP applied through nasal pillows and a nasal mask are equally effective in treating mild,

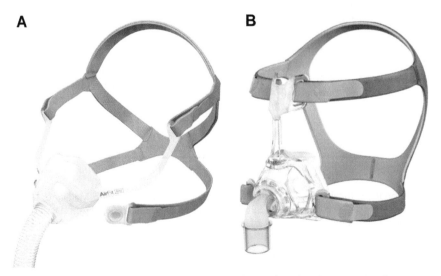

**Fig. 1.** Nasal masks. (*A*) N-10 and (*B*) Mirage FX by ResMed. (Reproduced with permission from ResMed. ResMed, Air10, Swift, Mirage are trademarks and/or registered trademarks of the ResMed family of companies.)

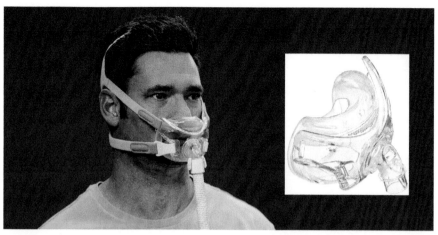

**Fig. 2.** Amara View. This interface uses a nasal cradle on top of a portion of the mask that covers the mouth. (*Courtesy of* Philips Respironics, Murrysville, PA.)

moderate, and severe sleep apnea.[6] A variety of nasal pillows are available; one major issue is finding the correct sized pillow (**Figs. 3** and **4**). Finding a mask with the proper pillow shape may require trying several brands of masks. Some models of nasal pillows are lighter, such as the Airfit P10 (ResMed, San Diego, CA), whereas others more stable, like the Swift LT (ResMed). Using too small a pillow size causes leak unless the mask is overtightened, which may cause nasal pain with prolonged use. In clinical practice, it has been found that, when patients are switched from a nasal mask to nasal pillows, they sometimes complain that the pressure feels much higher. This is due to the fact that the pressure drop across the nasal inlet is eliminated. Therefore, a slightly lower pressure may be needed when changing to nasal pillows.[7]

Nasal pillows may benefit patients by minimizing side effects such as claustrophobia, pressure sores, and air leak into the eyes.[8] They may also be useful in patients with mustaches or edentulous patients who have no dental support for the upper lip. A study by Zhu and colleagues[8] found that nasal pillows are as efficacious and subjectively as acceptable as nasal masks when treating OSA with high CPAP pressures. Therefore, one should not assume that nasal pillows will not work in patients on higher pressure. Nasal pillows are lighter and their initial acceptance might be higher; however, they can cause more nasal problems, particularly when a CPAP greater than 12 cm $H_2O$ is used.[3] Ryan and colleagues studied 21 patients with severe OSA using nasal masks and nasal pillows for 4 weeks each. The authors found no differences between the 2 types

**A**    **B**

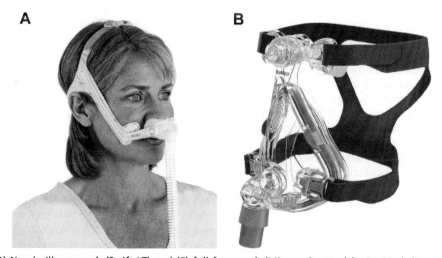

**Fig. 3.** (*A*) Nasal pillows mask (Swift LT) and (*B*) full face mask (Mirage Quattro) by ResMed. (Reproduced with permission from ResMed. ResMed, Air10, Swift, Mirage are trademarks and/or registered trademarks of the ResMed family of companies.)

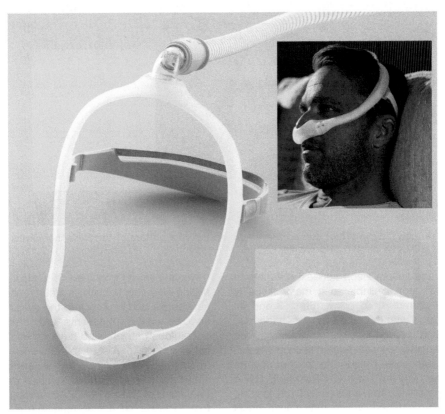

**Fig. 4.** DreamWear. This is a nasal cradle mask optimized to allow side sleeping. Airflow can enter from either side of the mask. (*Courtesy of* Philips Respironics, Murrysville, PA.)

of CPAP masks in terms of their impact on treatment adherence. However, the participants complained of nasal congestion, nasal dryness, nosebleeds, and headaches more frequently when they used nasal pillows than when they used nasal masks.[3] Use of adequate humidification, proper pillow size (avoiding the need for overtightening), and a saline gel may reduce potential problems with nasal pillows masks.

There are also specialty masks such as the total face mask, which covers the entire face including the eyes. The seal wraps around the outer most perimeter of the face. This moves the pressure off the cheeks and nose and may be an option for patients who have great difficulty obtaining an adequate seal with a nasal or oronasal mask. Oral interfaces (Oracle, Fisher Paykel, Auckland, New Zealand) are an option for patients with severe nasal congestion. However, dryness is a problem and the acceptance of oral interfaces is generally low (**Table 1**).

## GENERAL CONSIDERATIONS

Frequently, a trial of several masks is needed to find one that a patient can tolerate. Patients should

try different mask types in the sleep center before the start of a split or titration sleep study. Proper sizing and mask adjustment are crucial and should be checked at every clinic visit. It is important to ensure that mask fittings are performed properly because they are often done incorrectly. The mask is initially put on with the patient sitting upright; however, the straps should be adjusted while the patient is reclined because head position can affect mask tension. Some newer PAP devices have a check mask fit feature that gives the patient an estimate of mask fit before starting therapy. The machine attempts to do this by measuring the amount of leak. When trying on a new mask, it is essential to test the mask fit with the patient's treatment pressure to determine if the seal is adequate.

Patients tend to overtighten masks and this may actually impair the ability of the mask to seal properly. Adequate care and regular replacement of masks are paramount to maintain proper mask seal. Proper cleaning of the cushion with a gentle soap and water to remove facial oils may increase the lifespan of the membrane. Wiping the cushion with a damp cloth after each night may also be effective. With sleep onset, facial muscles relax

**Table 1**
**Different types of CPAP masks: advantages/disadvantages**

|  | Advantages/Indications | Disadvantages |
|---|---|---|
| Nasal pillows masks | Patients with claustrophobia<br>Intractable air leak into eyes with a nasal mask<br>Difficult obtaining a seal over upper nasal bridge with a nasal mask<br>No upper teeth or mustache makes obtaining a seal with a nasal mask difficult | Sensation of higher pressure in some patients<br>Nasal irritation (saline gel may help)<br>May not be tolerated in patients requiring high pressure |
| Oronasal masks | Patients with mouth leak or nasal congestion | Large area to obtain a seal (often associated with higher leak)<br>May be challenging in edentulous patients or those with facial creases<br>May worsen claustrophobia<br>May require higher treatment pressure than a nasal mask in some patients |
| Nasal masks | Smaller area to obtain a seal<br>In some patients, a lower pressure than needed with a full face mask may be effective | May require intervention for mouth leak (chin strap) or nasal congestion (medications and adequate humidification)<br>Air leak into eyes a potential problem |

(resulting in mouth opening or "jaw drop") and this slackening may change the ability of an oronasal mask to provide a good seal. In the case of intractable mouth leak owing to jaw drop, it may be necessary to use a larger size mask or wear a chin strap along with using an oronasal mask (under the mask).

## INTERVENTIONS FOR SIDE EFFECTS

Air leakage is a significant problem during CPAP therapy. It is experienced by up to 50% of nasal CPAP users and can cause a drop in mask pressure leading to suboptimal treatment, severe dryness, or repeated arousal from noise or eye irritation and these problems may result in poor compliance.[2] Oronasal masks are frequently used because of presumptive excessive mouth leak in some patients while using nasal masks.[9] Unintentional leaks may be caused by mouth opening or a poorly fitting mask. A disturbing leak may stem from air blowing toward the eyes and can also cause a disturbing noise (waking the patient or bed partner). Some leaks may occur only when PAP pressures are high. Some patients experience air leak when sleeping in the lateral position. The pillow under the head may push against the mask. "CPAP pillows" are available that have a recess on the side to prevent pressure against the mask.

Patients who breathe through their mouth either by habit or because of nasal obstruction.[3] In the presence of mouth leak, an early switch

from a nasal mask to an oronasal mask is a reasonable decision.[2] In 1 study of obese patients with OSA changing from a nasal to an oronasal mask, there was increased leak and residual apnea–hypopnea index; however, this did not affect the therapeutic pressure requirement.[10] Other studies suggest that a higher treatment pressure is required with oronasal compared with nasal masks.[5,11] A history of mouth breathing is not a clear contraindication to the use of nasal masks. There is evidence that the use of nasal CPAP leads to a change of habit, reducing mouth opening and the number of oral breaths. Some patients breathing through the nose and mouth while awake may switch to a nasal breathing route during sleep.[4] Use of a chin strap may be an effective intervention for mouth leak. In some individuals, intensive medical treatment of nasal congestion may allow a nasal interface to be used in a patient with difficulty breathing through the nose. Adequate humidification may also help to maintain nasal patency during the night. Drying of the nasal mucosa can increase nasal resistance.[12] Despite the potential problems with oronasal masks, many patients adapt well to them and exhibit good adherence and treatment efficacy.[3] Sometimes a mask leak with any interface will respond to a slight lowering of pressure. Also, switching from CPAP to an auto-PAP device may result in a lower mean nightly pressure and reduce leak.[7]

Claustrophobia is an important influential factor in CPAP adherence and an important clinical problem. Anxiety disorders are common among adults with OSA. Evidence suggests that anxiety disorders and the fear of choking may be more prevalent in severe OSA and in those adults with a higher body mass index.[13] Nasal pillow masks are often better tolerated compared with traditional nasal masks by patients with claustrophobia. Mask desensitization may also be an effective approach to reducing or eliminating claustrophobia in OSA treated with CPAP.[13] For patients with intractable mouth leak or mouth dryness who cannot tolerate an oronasal mask, they may prefer using a nasal mask with a chin strap (or a hybrid mask).

Facial pain related to CPAP, which may be described as dental or periodontal pain, is mainly caused by direct pressure of the device on the gums. This can occur in 15% to 20% of CPAP users.[14] In this case, nasal pillows may be better tolerated than nasal or oronasal masks. For skin irritation or a rash that develops from use of a PAP mask, there are CPAP mask liners that provide a soft layer between the face and CPAP mask cushion. The liner can help to prevent leaks and irritation while absorbing facial oils and moisture. Cloth PAP masks are also available and are made from a soft cloth, which can prevent pressure points from developing on the face during use. Gel nasal pads are available that can be placed across the nasal bridge and can help to reduce facial sores, minimize air leak into the eyes, and improve mask comfort.

Nasal congestion is a common symptom among PAP users. To manage nasal stuffiness, the cause should be treated and a mask change should be considered.[1] For dry or irritated nasal passages, which can be caused by the use of nasal pillows, the use of a saline nasal gel is recommended. If nasal congestion worsens over the night on PAP treatment, this is a clue that the patient may benefit from more humidification.

## ADJUNCTS TO MASKS

For patients who report entanglement of the CPAP hose during use of their machine, a hose caddy is a device that is used to lift the hose above the user while they are asleep. As mentioned, mask barriers such as CPAP mask liners act as a soft barrier between the silicone mask cushion and face. The liner can be used to prevent leaks and irritation around the cushion seal and protect skin from excessive moisture or residual red marks. To prevent skin irritation owing to the CPAP mask headstraps, there are

pads that slide over the lower strap of the CPAP mask headgear. As mentioned, patients who are side sleepers may find it difficult to keep the mask in place when they sleep in the lateral position. CPAP pillows are designed with contoured cutouts to prevent that mask from shifting toward 1 side of the face.

## REFERENCES

1. Bachour A, Vitikainen P, Maasilta P. Rates of initial acceptance of PAP masks and outcomes of mask switching. Sleep Breath 2016;20:733–8.
2. Neuzeret PC, Morin L. Impact of different nasal masks on CPAP therapy for obstructive sleep apnea: a randomized comparative trial. Clin Respir J 2016. [Epub ahead of print].
3. Andrade R, Piccin V, Nascimento J, et al. Impact of the type of mask on the effectiveness of and adherence to continuous positive airway pressure treatment for obstructive sleep apnea. J Bras Pneumol 2014;40:658–68.
4. Prosise GL, Berry RB. Oral-nasal continuous positive airway pressure as a treatment for obstructive sleep apnea. Chest 1994;106:180–6.
5. Ng JR, Aiyappan V, Mercer J, et al. Choosing an oronasal mask to deliver continuous positive airway pressure may cause more upper airway obstruction or lead to higher continuous positive airway pressure requirements than a nasal mask in some patients: a case series. J Clin Sleep Med 2016;12(9): 1227–32.
6. Ebben MR, Oyegbile T, Pollak CP. The efficacy of three different mask styles on a PAP titration night. Sleep Med 2012;13:645–9.
7. Berry RB, Wagner MH. Sleep medicine pearls. 3rd edition. Philadelphia: Saunders; 2014.
8. Zhu X, Wimms AJ, Benjafield AV. Assessment of the performance of nasal pillows at high CPAP pressures. J Clin Sleep Med 2013;9:873.
9. Bettinzoli M, Taranto-Montemurro L, Messineo L, et al. Oronasal masks require higher levels of positive airway pressure than nasal masks to treat obstructive sleep apnea. Sleep Breath 2014;18: 845–9.
10. Bakker JP, Neill AM, Campbell AJ. Nasal versus oronasal continuous positive airway pressure masks for obstructive sleep apnea: a pilot investigation of pressure requirement, residual disease, and leak. Sleep Breath 2012;16:709–16.
11. Deshpande S, Joosten S, Turton A, et al. Oronasal masks require a higher pressure than nasal and nasal pillow masks for the treatment of obstructive sleep apnea. J Clin Sleep Med 2016;12(9):1263–8.
12. Richard GL, Cistulli PA, Ugar G, et al. Mouth leak with nasal continuous positive airway pressure

increases nasal airway resistance. Am J Respir Crit Care Med 1996;154:182–6.

13. Edmonds JC, Yang H, King TS, et al. Claustrophobic tendencies and continuous positive airway pressure therapy non-adherence in adults with obstructive sleep apnea. Heart Lung 2015;44: 100–6.

14. Mermod M, Broome M, Hoarau R, et al. Facial pain associated with CPAP use: intra-sinusal third molar. Case Rep Otolaryngol 2014;2014:837252.

# Treatment of Obstructive Sleep Apnea

## Achieving Adherence to Positive Airway Pressure Treatment and Dealing with Complications

Christopher J. Lettieri, MD[a],[*], Scott G. Williams, MD[a],
Jacob F. Collen, MD[a], Emerson M. Wickwire, PhD[b],[c]

### KEYWORDS

- Obstructive sleep apnea • Positive airway pressure • Patient adherence
- Motivational enhancement therapy

### KEY POINTS

- Patient education and proactive support throughout the evaluation and treatment processes are the basis for maximal adherence.
- Pharmacologic and behavioral treatment of comorbid conditions, such as sinus congestion and insomnia, should be incorporated early in the treatment course or before initiating PAP.
- Multidisciplinary care teams are instrumental for achieving optimal patient care; members should include sleep medicine physicians, midlevel providers, behavioral specialists, and durable medical equipment support.
- Technical features of PAP platforms, including variable pressure delivery, expiratory pressure reductions, integrated humidification, and more advanced settings can improve patient comfort and enhance treatment effectiveness.
- Leveraging technology and implementing frequent follow-up assessments can help analyze patterns of PAP use and identify patients needing more intensive support or targeted adherence interventions.

## INTRODUCTION

Obstructive sleep apnea (OSA) is a common condition that is associated with multiple adverse consequences, including worsened health outcomes, diminished quality of life, and increased health care-related costs (**Box 1**).[1–3] The standard treatment for OSA is positive airway pressure (PAP), which has been in use since the early 1980s.[4,5] When used consistently, PAP therapy has been shown to reduce the negative health impact of many comorbid medical and psychiatric disorders.[6–8] Unfortunately, PAP adherence remains suboptimal.[9] Despite advances in both mask and PAP platform technology, which have incorporated multiple features to improve both comfort

Disclaimer: The views expressed in this review reflect those of the authors, and do not constitute official policy of the United States Army or Department of Defense.
[a] Department of Pulmonary, Critical Care, and Sleep Medicine, Walter Reed National Military Medical Center, 8901 Wisconsin Avenue, Bethesda, MD 20889, USA; [b] Department of Psychiatry, University of Maryland School of Medicine, 100 North Greene Street, 2nd Floor, Baltimore, MD 21201, USA; [c] Sleep Disorders Center, Division of Pulmonary and Critical Care Medicine, Department of Medicine, University of Maryland School of Medicine, 100 North Greene Street, 2nd Floor, Baltimore, MD 21201, USA
* Corresponding author.
*E-mail address:* christopher.j.lettieri.mil@mail.mil

Sleep Med Clin 12 (2017) 551–564
http://dx.doi.org/10.1016/j.jsmc.2017.07.005
1556-407X/17/Published by Elsevier Inc.

sleep.theclinics.com

> **Box 1**
> **Complications of positive airway pressure**
>
> Mask interface problems
>   Skin irritation
>   Skin breakdown
>   Change in dentitions
>   Mask discomfort
> Claustrophobia
> Vasomotor rhinitis
> Transient insomnia
> Dry mouth
> Aerophagia
> Central or complex sleep apnea

and the effective delivery of pressure, adherence has not improved substantially.

By any measure, the optimal treatment of OSA requires long-term behavior changes, which include sleep habits, diet and exercise, and adherence with therapeutic interventions. Poor adoption is evident throughout the continuum of care. This is particularly true of PAP. Whether this lack of adherence is unique to PAP, or reflects multiple overlapping confounders and merely highlighted because this therapy includes integrated objective measures of use, remains a source on ongoing debate. Regardless, both acceptance of and adherence to PAP therapy remains problematic. For example, up to 30% of patients fail to initiate therapy after diagnosis.[10] Of those starting therapy, approximately 25% stop within the first year, and fewer than 50% remain adherent in the long term.[11–14] Even among those who use CPAP regularly, average nighttime use is only 3.5 to 5.3 hours.[15–17]

Despite these challenges, several interventions have been shown to improve PAP use and, subsequently, improve patient outcomes. The purpose of this review is to define PAP adherence, identify and discuss current challenges faced by clinicians as they provide PAP therapy to their patients, and provide an overview of the various strategies to increase PAP use, with an emphasis on understanding, recognizing, and overcoming common barriers to care and using high-yield interventions early in the treatment course.

## QUANTIFYING ADHERENCE WITH POSITIVE AIRWAY PRESSURE TREATMENT

Currently accepted insurance criteria in the United States contend that "adherent" equates to the use of PAP greater than 4 hours per night for at least 70% of nights.[15,18] Therefore, an individual only has to use PAP 86 hours per month, or 35% of the total recommended sleep time, to be considered adherent. Although many argue that this definition of adherence is grossly insufficient and most likely contributes to the limited ability of PAP to resolve both symptoms and consequences associated with OSA, the fact remains that despite using a low threshold for adherence, most patients do not achieve it. PAP use is commonly measured objectively. Although objective measures are intuitively superior to subjective reports, they do not always reflect the entire history. For PAP, adherence reports reveal the amount of time the PAP device was in use. They do not include time spent awake, nor do they record sleep without PAP. As such, they can both overestimate and underestimate sleep. In addition, these reports do not differentiate between patients who only intermittently use PAP, those who use it every night but only for part of the night, or those who use PAP during every sleep period but are grossly sleep restricted. As a result, commonly reported objective measures represent an upperbound estimate of how long PAP was worn during sleep, which is frequently an inaccurate reflection of both total sleep time and true adherence. All of these possibilities can be attributed to the persistence of symptoms, with significant variability regarding the effectiveness of PAP between each of these three scenarios. In other words, the persistence of symptoms may reflect insufficient sleep, insufficient use of PAP, limitations in the efficacy of PAP, or some combination of each. And, despite their objective nature, PAP use reports do not answer this question. Clinical assessment and results of PAP outcomes research should be interpreted with this limitation in mind.

Regardless of the limitations related to the accuracy of how PAP use is measured, there is sufficient evidence regarding the efficacy of PAP. And, it is clear that increased use leads to greater improvements in outcomes. In short, this therapy is efficacious, but its effectiveness is limited by insufficient use. Multiple studies have reported a dose–response relationship between hours of PAP use and improvements in OSA severity,[19] neurocognitive performance,[20] symptoms, and mortality.[21] Some outcomes have been shown to improve with even limited PAP use, and some seem to have a ceiling effect, where additional use may not lead to further improvements. This circumstance has contributed to the low threshold defining PAP adherence. However, improvements in other outcomes are not observed unless PAP is used for more than 6 or 7 hours per night. For example, a 2007 study by Weaver and colleagues[22] showed that, depending on the outcome, different durations of nightly PAP use were required to show improvement. Subjective alertness improved after 4 hours of use, whereas objective improvements in mean sleep latency required at least 6 hours, and functional outcomes required at least 7 hours of PAP use per night for optimization. Similarly, Antic and colleagues[23] reported a variable dose response for changes in subjective and objective somnolence, as well as improvements in neurobehavioral assessments.

Unfortunately, many studies do not report the dose response to PAP therapy, so it is challenging to define the beneficial impact of "optimal" use. As an example, a recent study considered the effect of PAP therapy on resistant hypertension and found that PAP resulted in a significant decrease in systolic blood pressure (3.08 mm Hg; 95% CI, 1.79–4.37), diastolic blood pressure (2.28 mm Hg; 95% CI, 1.56–3.00), and mean arterial pressure (2.54 mm Hg; 95% CI, 1.73–3.36) within the first year of treatment.[24] This effect size is less than a typical antihypertensive.[25] However, this study did not stratify PAP users by hours of therapy per night, or regular use. Thus, it was impossible to discern the optimal duration of PAP use in this sample. Nonetheless, in a clinical context, we recommend that patients are advised to wear PAP during all sleep periods.

## WHAT FACTORS AFFECT ADHERENCE TO POSITIVE AIRWAY PRESSURE TREATMENT?

A number of factors have been identified that influence both acceptance of and adherence to PAP therapy. More easily measured factors relate to demographic, physiologic, and disease-specific variables. Perhaps more important, the influence of a patient's understanding of the underlying disorder and therapeutic strategy, their perceived benefit of treatment, their initial experiences with an intervention, and their overall health behaviors are becoming increasingly recognized as impactful determinants of both therapeutic adherence and outcomes.

Several variables regarding patient demographics, such as age, gender, ethnicity, socioeconomic status, and education level, have been shown to influence PAP adherence, although with variable results.[13,26–32] The impact of disease-specific features, such as OSA severity, degree of symptoms, and presence of medical comorbidities, are similarly inconsistent.[13,26–28,33] Although more well-defined markers of OSA severity have not always been shown to influence adherence, certain physiologic factors, such as increased nasal resistance and claustrophobia, are clearly associated with increased difficulty in adapting to PAP and represent modifiable risk factors for adherence.[34,35]

Both the perceived benefit of, and subjective response to, therapy represent the most robust determinants of PAP adherence. Adherence requires that a patient perceive the treatment as being beneficial, be motivated to initiate therapy, and have a sense of self-efficacy regarding the use of PAP.[36] Self-efficacy, or a patient's belief that they can use PAP successfully, is a modifiable psychological variable that is consistently related to PAP adherence.[37] Patients who lack a sense of motivation or perceived benefit, or those who endorse negative perceptions regarding inconvenience or discomfort with PAP, are not likely to use therapy. The patient's understanding of the underlying condition, the consequences of remaining untreated, and the available therapies and their benefits substantially influence these perceptions. These understandings can be enhanced through education and an individualized approach to therapeutic decisions.

A patient's understanding of OSA and benefits of PAP will not improve adherence in isolation. Although their perception of how PAP will benefit them can greatly influence acceptance of PAP, their response to therapy greatly influences their continued use of PAP. Although baseline symptoms have been shown to predict subsequent PAP use, adherence is significantly higher among those who experience greater reductions of these symptoms. Those who are more symptomatic have the potential of perceiving more symptomatic improvements. Equally important, those who have more comfort and a better initial experience with PAP are more likely to continue use, and early experiences with PAP predict long-term use.[27,38,39] This can be achieved by addressing 2 fundamental aspects in initiating PAP therapy. First, clinicians must identify and overcome common conditions, as explained elsewhere in this article, that can reduce the initial comfort and tolerance of PAP. Second, the initial PAP settings must optimize both comfort and the ablation of obstructive events. The quality of the PAP titration can impact subsequent compliance and persistent sleep apnea will quickly lead to a poor perception regarding the benefits of therapy.[40] Thus, it is imperative that clinicians adopt a proactive approach toward PAP adherence and seek to identify facilitators and barriers to PAP use as early as possible. Early impressions are critical, and a patient's attitude toward treatment and initial experiences can predict subsequent use.[41] Indeed, psychological instruments assessing subjective well-being and health status were able to correctly predict 85.7% of nonadherent patients in 1 study.[42]

In our clinical experience, PAP adherence and other health-related behaviors are frequently correlated. Medication nonadherence, inconsistent bedtimes,[43] smoking, alcohol use, and other unhealthy behaviors may be markers for both poor adherence and a reduced therapeutic response.[44,45] We found that PAP use paralleled medications adherence.[46] Although it is well-shown that PAP use remains problematic, it may not be unique to this specific treatment, but rather reflect an overall poor adherence with medical therapies and healthy behaviors, which is only recognized and highlighted because PAP includes objective measures of use. Regardless, these behaviors reflect, and can help to identify patients at an increased risk for PAP nonadherence.

As presented, there are numerous factors that can negatively impact PAP adherence. However, these also represent both a means to identify high-risk patients and potential targets for intervention. Although a multitude of interventions aimed to improve PAP use have been studied, they each require additional costs and resources. Given the increasing prevalence of OSA, it would be prohibitive to apply all interventions to all patients. Recognizing those at an increased risk for poor adherence or discontinuation of PAP can help to focus the correct intervention toward the correct patient to individualize care and maximize the benefits of therapy.

## COMMON BARRIERS TO ADHERENCE TO POSITIVE AIRWAY PRESSURE TREATMENT AND HOW TO OVERCOME THEM

Initial experience with PAP predicts long-term use, so potential barriers to adherence should be addressed early and readdressed on an ongoing basis.[19,27,40] A proactive clinical approach is particularly important, because many new PAP users report side effects during the acclimatization phase of therapy.[47] Common complaints impacting adherence are sinus congestion, mask discomfort, insomnia, and claustrophobia. Early assessment and intervention may improve adherence and long-term patient outcomes.

Intolerance of the mask interface is the most common complaint leading to PAP discontinuation or exploration of other, non-PAP treatments for OSA. Several studies have evaluated the impact of mask type on PAP adherence. Although the type of mask interface is often considered interchangeable, the available literature suggests that nasal masks may provide better patient acceptance and comfort, lower required pressure and residual apnea–hypopnea index (AHI), and fewer side effects compared with other mask types.[48–53] Oronasal masks may induce anatomic obstruction by pushing the tongue posteriorly[54] and studies have noted that these masks are associated with increased pressure requirements, higher residual AHIs, and lower rates of adherence compared with nasal masks.[48,55–59] The importance of proper mask selection and sizing cannot be overemphasized and can frequently mitigate this common barrier to PAP use. When PAP therapy is initiated, patients should have a formal custom mask fitting and assistance with mask selection by a specially trained respiratory therapist. Patients should be educated about proper fit, donning, and care of their mask. Many patients are unaware that masks should be periodically replaced. Over time, the mask liner deteriorates, resulting in skin irritation and leak, and potentially promoting patient discomfort and poor adherence.

Nasal congestion is both a frequent complaint among patients with OSA and is a common barrier to PAP use. Up to 14% of the US population has chronic sinus disease, with an even higher proportion experiencing acute allergic flares.[60] This prevalence is significantly higher among patients with OSA, with 40% reporting chronic rhinitis. Sinus congestion is a common cause of PAP discomfort and decreases its efficacy. As such, it is important to recognize and treat before initiating PAP. Not only is preexisting nasal congestion common among those with OSA, it can also occur as a result of PAP therapy, typically early in the course of treatment. As many as 30% of patients report developing nasal congestion during the initial weeks of therapy, with 10% having persistent symptoms for several months.[61] PAP-induced vasomotor rhinitis occurs as a dose–response phenomenon, with higher pressures causing more significant symptoms.[62] Heated, humidified air can reduce congestion,[63] and this consequence of PAP use has greatly decreased with wide adaptation of integrated humidifiers in most PAP platforms. However, nasal steroids or nasal antimuscarinics may be required for those who develop nasal congestion despite the use of a humidifier.

Comorbid insomnia occurs in up to 55% of patients with OSA and a bidirectional relationship between insomnia and OSA has been postulated.[64] Clinical experience suggests that, when insomnia is caused by sleep fragmentation arising from intermittent airway obstruction, symptoms frequently resolve with PAP therapy.[65–67] However, the existence of both sleep initiation and maintenance insomnia pose significant barriers to PAP use, and adapting to therapy can often prove challenging and cause further difficulties with sleep onset and continuity.[68] Similarly, insomnia-related posttraumatic stress disorder has been shown to both worsen OSA-related symptoms and quality of life measures, but also significantly reduces the use of and response to PAP.[69–71] A brief course of sedative-hypnotics may assist with the initial adaptation of PAP for those with preexisting insomnia.[72] However, nonpharmacologic therapy is the preferred treatment for insomnia, including for those with comorbid OSA, and the National Institutes of Health, American Academy of Sleep Medicine, and American College of Physicians all recommend cognitive-behavioral treatment for insomnia as first-line treatment for chronic insomnia, including insomnia occurring in the context of other medical, psychiatric, or sleep disorders.[73–75] In patients with OSA, CBT for insomnia has been shown to improve tolerance, effectiveness, and patient satisfaction with PAP.[76]

PAP-induced anxiety and claustrophobia can also present substantial barriers to therapy.[77] Even after proper mask selection and fitting, a subset of patients continues to describe difficulty sleeping with the mask interface. Although sometimes confused with insomnia, claustrophobia is a very different barrier and can be treated with simple desensitization in most cases. For persistent symptoms, referral to a behavioral sleep medicine specialist is often very helpful in these instances.[78] Use of an abbreviated daytime polysomnogram (ie, "PAP NAP") may also facilitate accommodation to PAP therapy and improve adherence.[79]

## ADDITIONAL NONPHARMACOLOGIC INTERVENTIONS TO IMPROVE ADHERENCE TO POSITIVE AIRWAY PRESSURE TREATMENT
### Education

Successful treatment with PAP starts with a comprehensive patient education plan. The decision to use PAP, like any medical treatment, involves both a commitment and associated lifestyle changes. It is important to realize that the treating clinician is asking the patient to change the way they sleep every single night. This means that one-third of their lives will be directly altered by this decision. And, the transition to PAP therapy may initially worsen their sleep. Education must be an ongoing process, starting from the initial assessment and continuing at every patient encounter. And, it must extend beyond OSA and PAP and include information regarding sleep

health, proper sleep habits, and the benefits of resolving sleep disorders. Although this might seem like common sense and can significantly improve outcomes, thorough patient education is, unfortunately, not common practice. A recent trial randomizing patients to either simply reviewing the results of their polysomnogram with a clinician or not found, not surprisingly, that those who spoke with sleep medicine staff and understood the importance of treating sleep-disordered breathing had significantly greater PAP use.[80]

Numerous studies have evaluated a range of programs, including video-education protocols,[81,82] patient education literature,[83] small group problem-based learning,[84] and CBT. Although improvements in adherence for some programs have been inconsistent,[36,83,85,86] programs using CBT (including desensitization, CBT for insomnia, and motivational enhancement [ME]) have been largely effective.[87–92] Unfortunately, these programs require a significant amount of time and expertise, and may not feasible in all practices.

The importance of spousal involvement for optimizing patient outcomes cannot be overstated. However, there is little high-quality objective evidence to discern the exact contribution of bed partner involvement in care. In a recent review, Ye and colleagues[93] considered the qualitative nature of the bed partner dynamic. Of 30 studies included in the most recent Cochrane review of behavioral interventions to improve PAP adherence, only 2 included the spouses of patients with OSA.[94] Given that the most common impetus for referral to a sleep facility is bed partner complaint, and considering patients frequently report potential PAP-induced spousal sleep disturbances as a primary excuses not to use therapy,[95] it is critical to include them in the education and treatment plan.[96] Clinical experience suggests that inclusion of bed partners and family members in routine clinical care can produce dramatic results. One study comparing those who slept alone with those with a consistent bed partner found PAP use increased 1.3 hours per night if a bed partner was present.[39] In another study, PAP was used more often during nights when married couples slept in the same bed.[97] It is essential, therefore, to educate patients that PAP tends to improve sleep quality for both patients and spouses.[98–100]

Group appointments can offer additional benefits related to PAP adherence. Not only do they reduce per-patient resources, they also provide less tangible benefits such as a shared sense of purpose and bonding over a common experience. Brostrom and colleagues[84] used a problem-based learning small group tutorial to improve PAP adherence in 25 subjects. After this educational program, 72% were adherent with PAP, with persistent benefits noted 6 months later.[84] In contrast, Basoglu and colleagues[81] failed to find a benefit from the addition of an educational video compared with standard physician instructions alone. We previously published the benefits of a comprehensive group educational program during PAP initiation.[101] Compared with individual counseling, group education led to both improved adherence and a 3-to 4-fold increase in access to care. The benefits of patient education and improved outcomes are well-established, and group education strategies may be a useful option for clinics that lack the resources to provide intensive education on an individual basis.

## Motivational Enhancement

Motivational interviewing and ME are patient-centered psychological approaches that have demonstrated effectiveness for improving patient adherence in conditions ranging from cardiovascular disease and diabetes to nutrition and substance use disorders.[102] Multiple authors have found positive results from ME-based interventions among patients with OSA.[87,91,103–105] Although most of the ME research in the OSA population has been conducted by the same group, there is a consistent trend toward positive results.[87] In 2007, Aloia and colleagues[103] compared standard education, ME, and a control group. The probability of PAP discontinuation in the control group was 51%, compared with 30% in the education group and 26% in the ME group. Although the probability of reaching adherence was not significant different (61% control group, 68% education group, 67% ME group). Although ME might not significantly improve adherence, it may help to identify those who will discontinue therapy and allow clinics to manage these patients differently. This study was followed by a recent paper in which individual at greater risk did demonstrate a 97-minute per night increase after ME compared with controls.[104] Although behavioral treatments are often considered a "fix" for poor adherence, we believe that patient motivation is an essential aspect of OSA care. One of the key features of ME is that it is useful only if the patient desires to make a change. Therefore, identifying motivated patients before PAP initiation is critical to maximizing the success of ME and help to prioritize and appropriately allocate other resources intended to promote adherence.

## Telehealth and Technology

As a result of technological advancements, PAP automated tracking technologies offer the opportunity to improve medical care for patients with OSA that is unlike the monitoring capabilities we have for most other chronic diseases. Historically, these technologies have provided clinicians with data on how much the patient is using PAP, how effective it is (based on indirect measurements of airflow limitation, which are interpreted as a residual AHI), and mask leak (which may indicate mask fit and comfort). The 2013 American Thoracic Society guidance for interpreting PAP compliance reports recommends a cutoff value for the residual AHI of fewer than 10 events per hour as indicative of satisfactory control of OSA.[106] It should be noted that a high residual AHI may lead to persistence of symptoms, poor sleep quality, and a loss of confidence in the value of PAP, and subsequently lead to its discontinuation by patients. As such, this threshold may be too high for most patients and it is recommended to optimize the ablation of obstructive events to promote better outcomes and adherence.

Heated humidification is a comfort feature that is felt to improve adherence, potentially by reducing symptoms of dry mouth and nasal congestion. The available literature suggests that there is little evidence that heated humidification provides substantial or clinically significant benefits for PAP adherence and a systematic Cochrane review found little impact on compliance.[107,108] However, humidification can mitigate some discomfort with PAP therapy, particularly oronasal dryness. Further, 1 study demonstrated that heated humidification could increase PAP use by 36 minutes per night.[95] Nonetheless, we provide heated humidification to all our patients. Our clinical experience is that most patients derive benefit from the heated humidification, either from comfort, or from having a sense of control in adjusting the setting on their appliance.

Transient and synchronized flexible alterations in the delivered pressure during both the inspiratory and expiratory portions of the respiratory phase has become a common feature in most PAP platforms, and is intended to improve comfort and tolerability to improve adherence. Although similar in design, each manufacturer uses its own patented technology: for example, ResMed (ResMed Corp, San Diego, CA) uses EPR and Philips-Respironics (Koninklijke Philips Electronics, NV, Eindhoven, the Netherlands) use A-Flex or C-Flex. There are few data in the published literature regarding the impact that these technologies have on PAP adherence.[36] Aloia and colleagues[109] found that C-Flex improved adherence compared with standard CPAP. However, there were no differences noted in symptomatic improvement. Chihara and colleagues[110] compared the impact on adherence between standard APAP, APAP plus C-Flex, and APAP plus A-Flex. The investigators demonstrated that C-Flex was superior to both standard APAP and APAP plus A-Flex. Although these features can improve comfort, they largely have not shown benefit in significantly improving PAP use or adherence. In addition, the changes in pressure can lead to sleep fragmentation and the reduced pressure during exhalation may result in instability of the airways and a persistence of apneic events. Ultimately, more studies are needed to evaluate the impact of these technologies on adherence.

## PHARMACOLOGIC INTERVENTIONS TO IMPROVE ADHERENCE TO POSITIVE AIRWAY PRESSURE TREATMENT

Sedative hypnotics, in particular nonbenzodiazepine receptor agonists (NBRAs), offer an attractive option for improving adherence, particularly when used during the initial experiences with PAP. NBRAs do not adversely impact the AHI, oxygen saturation ($SpO_2$), sleep architecture, or response to PAP therapy.[111–113] The use of a sedative hypnotic during initial polysomnography has been shown to improve adherence, likely by facilitating a more accurate pressure determination and by improving the initial experience with PAP.[114–117] Similarly, the transient use of these agents should improve the transition to PAP therapy. However, studies assessing the usefulness of NBRAs for improving the transition to PAP therapy have had mixed results. In a study by Bradshaw and colleagues,[112] zolpidem failed to demonstrate a benefit on improving PAP compliance. In contrast, we found that 2 weeks of eszopiclone during PAP initiation led to more PAP use, less PAP discontinuation, and a greater likelihood of achieving adherence compared with placebo.[72] Eszopiclone has a longer duration of action than zolpidem, facilitating increased sleep continuity, which may explain the differences noted in these studies. Although most studies have evaluated nonselected patients with OSA, it is likely that the greatest benefit of NBRAs is for patients with comorbid insomnia.[36,118] Given that insomnia is a substantial barrier to PAP acceptance, means to facilitate the transition to therapy are needed to prevent abandonment of treatment.

Not only do sedatives have a role in aiding in the initial transition of PAP therapy, they may be beneficial in the management of sleep-disordered breathing. There is increasing recognition regarding the arousal threshold in sleep apnea, and patients with a low arousal threshold may represent a unique phenotype of OSA. In these individuals, airflow limitations may lead to sleep fragmentation in the absence of significant gas exchange abnormalities, possibly owing to sensitivity to the degree of stimuli required to cause an arousal or awakening.[119,120] Both trazodone and eszopiclone have been shown to improve the AHI and sleep continuity in patients with the low arousal threshold phenotype, and may provide a mechanism for improving adherence and outcomes.[119] However, these potential benefits need to be weighed against the effects of long-term use of sedatives.

## COMPLICATIONS OF POSITIVE AIRWAY PRESSURE THERAPY AND HOW TO PREVENT OR OVERCOME THEM

Although safe and typically well-tolerated, there are several potential complications of PAP therapy, in addition to vasomotor rhinitis already discussed, that may have a negative impact on adherence. Proper patient education may mitigate the development of many of these complications. In addition, patients should be queried regarding their occurrence during each follow-up visit to promptly recognize and treat them to minimize their effect on PAP tolerance.

Aerophagia may result from positive pressure therapy. Patients may experience reflux, belching, distension, cramping, flatulence, and generalized gastrointestinal discomfort. Aerophagia is a challenging topic for clinicians, with limited evidence to guide management. Two physiologic mechanisms may contribute to this phenomenon. Air that enters the oropharynx under positive pressure may be swallowed and misdirected to the esophagus. Swallowed air can contribute to lower esophageal relaxation and cause or worsen reflux and nocturnal symptoms of gastroesophageal reflux disease.[121–123] Swallowed air can also trigger a reflexive closure of the upper esophageal sphincter, preventing escape of air, which can lead to abdominal distention and flatulence. Aerophagia is more common in patients with gastroesophageal reflux disease and those on antireflux medication. It also occurs more commonly in those with chronic sinus congestion, likely owing to an increase in upper airway resistance. In addition, hyperflexion of the neck from pillows can lead to partial closure of the upper airways, facilitating air to enter the esophagus instead of the trachea. By routine and unless otherwise contraindicated, we advise all patients with OSA to elevate the head of their beds 4 to 6 inches and use only a single, flat pillow to minimize this occurrence. In addition, we recommend treatment of sinus congestion before initiation of PAP to both reduce the development of aerophagia and to address this common barrier to PAP tolerability, as discussed. For patients using an oronasal mask interface who develop aerophagia, switching to a nasal mask may resolve this. Compared with full-face masks, nasal masks produce a relatively greater negative pressure gradient in the posterior oropharynx that, in theory, should result in less air swallowing. When these techniques are unsuccessful, clinicians may elect to reduce the prescribed PAP pressure. Although there is no literature supporting pressure change as an avenue to improve aerophagia, anecdotal experiences have fund this to be beneficial in some patients. However, this should be balanced with the potential for inadequately treated OSA. Ultimately, patients with ongoing complaints should be referred to a gastroenterologist to assess for hiatal hernia or other conditions outside the scope of a sleep physician that may be causing these symptoms.

Central apneas and periodic breathing may occur in patients with OSA following the initiation of PAP therapy. "Treatment-emergent" or "complex" sleep apnea develops in up to 19% of patients. In the majority of cases, these central events resolve with continued PAP use, likely owing to normalization of $Pco_2$ and the hypercarbic threshold. However, 5% to 26% of patients will have persistent (>3 months) complex sleep apnea.[124] This condition highlights the multitude of physiologic underpinnings of sleep-disordered breathing, with upper airway collapsibility promoting obstructive events, and correction of airway tone with PAP promoting central apneas and an unstable respiratory pattern owing to increased chemosensitivity, low arousal threshold, and increased loop gain. Conservative measures, including optimization of heart failure therapies when indicated, weight loss, improved sleep hygiene, and reducing use of opioid medications, may alleviate the condition, to a degree. Non-PAP medical therapies, such as sedatives to increase the arousal threshold (decrease the number of arousals), respiratory stimulants such as acetazolamide, inhaled $CO_2$, addition of dead-space ventilation, and supplemental oxygen, are often less feasible owing to cost, difficult implementation, lack of availability or expertise, and limited empiric evidence.[125] When identified, the continued use of CPAP with close observation is the first option for most practitioners and, as stated, resolution of central events occurs in most patients after several weeks on PAP therapy.[125] Patients with persistent complex sleep apnea can be treated with biphasic PAP or adaptive servo-ventilation (ASV). ASV is well-tolerated by most patients and will resolve central apneas and periodic breathing faster and more effectively than CPAP, especially in the short term.[124,126] Deciding whether to use a watchful waiting approach with continued CPAP, or adopting ASV early in the course of treatment depends on many considerations, including cost and how quickly a treatment response is needed.[125] Because PAP adherence is determined early, a more conservative strategy with CPAP may lead some patients to abandon therapy. Our practice is to provide close clinical follow-up and consider ASV in those whose central events do not resolve with CPAP. Given the recent results of SERVE-HF, we avoid the use of ASV in patients with a left ventricular ejection fraction of less than or equal to 45%.[127]

Local complications resulting from mask interfaces include skin irritation, visible indentations that are cosmetically unappealing, and skin ulceration in regions of maximal contact (ie, nasal bridge).[128] Eye irritation and keratitis from mask leak have also been reported. Often, these events can be resolved or even prevented with proper mask selection and educating patients on the proper way to don and adjust the mask. Patients often overtighten masks to resolve air leaks. This overtightening is not only counterproductive in most cases, it can also cause or contribute to skin ulcerations. Proper mask selection and sizing that is both compatible with the patient's facial features and pressure requirements and minimized air leak is crucial because this measure will enhance comfort and efficacy while also reducing complications. Several lotions and barriers intended to reduce mask-induced skin irritation and ulceration are commercially available; however, no clinical data are available to assess their usefulness.

Craniofacial changes and alterations in bite occlusion may occur with PAP, particularly among those using nasal masks. In a prospective study assessing craniofacial changes after 2 years of PAP use, Tsuda and coworkers[129] found that nasal CPAP led to significant retrusion of the anterior maxilla, a setback of the chin positions, a subluxation of the maxillary incisors, and bite malocclusion.

## SUMMARY

PAP remains the most efficacious treatment for OSA and is the first choice of treatment for most patients. However, challenges with adherence remain problematic. Numerous trials show improved subjective and objective outcomes from successfully treating OSA. In contrast, several studies have failed to observe that PAP significantly improves symptoms or end-organ dysfunction. However, these studies are largely limited by insufficient use of therapy. The fact remains that PAP only works if it is being used. And, despite the barriers to PAP use, the majority of motivated patients can become adherent. If clinicians adopt a comprehensive strategy to systematically assess and remedy barriers to care, the likelihood of optimal treatment dramatically increases. We recommend a patient-centered, stepwise approach to maximizing PAP adherence (**Fig. 1**). We also recommend that patients failing to achieve adherence with PAP should receive a retrial of therapy using these strategies. For patients who continue to refuse or are intolerant of therapy, alternatives to PAP, particularly oral appliances, should be used as the primary objective is to ensure their OA is sufficiently treated.

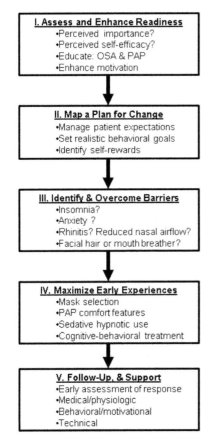

**Fig. 1.** A patient-centered, stepwise approach to maximizing adherence to positive airway pressure (PAP) treatment. From a motivational perspective, patients must be ready to attempt PAP. Clinicians and care teams should provide comprehensive disease education including not only personalized consequences of obstructive sleep apnea (OSA) and potential health benefits of treatment, but also patient-centered and patient-defined improvements in quality of life that might result from treatment. Next, patient expectations should be managed, and a detailed care plan with deadline and rewards for adherence should be established. Potential barriers to PAP adherence such as insomnia or rhinitis should be identified and addressed as early in the treatment plan as possible. Early experiences are essential to long-term PAP success, and clinicians and care teams should strive to "front-load" support to patients and family members. Finally, ongoing follow-up with attention to medical, physiologic, behavioral, motivational, and technical factors is essential. (*From* Wickwire EM, Lettieri CJ, Cairns AA, et al. Maximizing positive airway pressure adherence in adults: a common-sense approach. Chest 2013;144(2):689; with permission.)

## REFERENCES

1. Punjabi NM, Shahar E, Redline S, et al. Sleep-disordered breathing, glucose intolerance, and insulin resistance: the Sleep Heart Health Study. Am J Epidemiol 2004;160(6):521–30.
2. Shahar E, Whitney CW, Redline S, et al. Sleep-disordered breathing and cardiovascular disease: cross-sectional results of the Sleep Heart Health Study. Am J Respir Crit Care Med 2001;163(1):19–25.
3. Shepard JW Jr. Hypertension, cardiac arrhythmias, myocardial infarction, and stroke in relation to obstructive sleep apnea. Clin Chest Med 1992;13(3):437–58.
4. Kushida CA, Littner MR, Hirshkowitz M, et al. Practice parameters for the use of continuous and bilevel positive airway pressure devices to treat adult patients with sleep-related breathing disorders. Sleep 2006;29(3):375–80.
5. Sullivan CE, Issa FG, Berthon-Jones M, et al. Reversal of obstructive sleep apnoea by continuous positive airway pressure applied through the nares. Lancet 1981;1(8225):862–5.
6. Guo J, Sun Y, Xue LJ, et al. Effect of CPAP therapy on cardiovascular events and mortality in patients with obstructive sleep apnea: a meta-analysis. Sleep Breath 2016;20(3):965–74.
7. Montserrat JM, Ferrer M, Hernandez L, et al. Effectiveness of CPAP treatment in daytime function in sleep apnea syndrome: a randomized controlled study with an optimized placebo. Am J Respir Crit Care Med 2001;164(4):608–13.
8. Sanchez AI, Buela-Casal G, Bermudez MP, et al. The effects of continuous positive air pressure treatment on anxiety and depression levels in apnea patients. Psychiatry Clin Neurosci 2001;55(6):641–6.
9. Weaver TE, Grunstein RR. Adherence to continuous positive airway pressure therapy: the challenge to effective treatment. Proc Am Thorac Soc 2008;5(2):173–8.

10. Collard P, Pieters T, Aubert G, et al. Compliance with nasal CPAP in obstructive sleep apnea patients. Sleep Med Rev 1997;1(1):33–44.

11. Edinger JD, Carwile S, Miller P, et al. Psychological status, syndromatic measures, and compliance with nasal CPAP therapy for sleep apnea. Percept Mot Skills 1994;78(3 Pt 2):1116–8.

12. Marquez-Baez C, Paniagua-Soto J, Castilla-Garrido JM. Treatment of sleep apnea syndrome with CPAP: compliance with treatment, its efficacy and secondary effects. Rev Neurol 1998;26(151):375–80 [in Spanish].

13. McArdle N, Devereux G, Heidarnejad H, et al. Long-term use of CPAP therapy for sleep apnea/hypopnea syndrome. Am J Respir Crit Care Med 1999;159(4 Pt 1):1108–14.

14. Pepin JL, Krieger J, Rodenstein D, et al. Effective compliance during the first 3 months of continuous positive airway pressure. A European prospective study of 121 patients. Am J Respir Crit Care Med 1999;160(4):1124–9.

15. Kribbs NB, Pack AI, Kline LR, et al. Objective measurement of patterns of nasal CPAP use by patients with obstructive sleep apnea. Am Rev Respir Dis 1993;147(4):887–95.

16. Loube DI, Gay PC, Strohl KP, et al. Indications for positive airway pressure treatment of adult obstructive sleep apnea patients: a consensus statement. Chest 1999;115(3):863–6.

17. Reeves-Hoche MK, Meck R, Zwillich CW. Nasal CPAP: an objective evaluation of patient compliance. Am J Respir Crit Care Med 1994;149(1):149–54.

18. Brown LK. Use it or lose it: Medicare's new paradigm for durable medical equipment coverage? Chest 2010;138(4):785–9.

19. Stepnowsky CJ, Dimsdale JE. Dose-response relationship between CPAP compliance and measures of sleep apnea severity. Sleep Med 2002;3(4):329–34.

20. Zimmerman ME, Arnedt JT, Stanchina M, et al. Normalization of memory performance and positive airway pressure adherence in memory-impaired patients with obstructive sleep apnea. Chest 2006;130(6):1772–8.

21. Campos-Rodriguez F, Pena-Grinan N, Reyes-Nunez N, et al. Mortality in obstructive sleep apnea-hypopnea patients treated with positive airway pressure. Chest 2005;128(2):624–33.

22. Weaver TE, Maislin G, Dinges DF, et al. Relationship between hours of CPAP use and achieving normal levels of sleepiness and daily functioning. Sleep 2007;30(6):711–9.

23. Antic NA, Catcheside P, Buchan C, et al. The effect of CPAP in normalizing daytime sleepiness, quality of life, and neurocognitive function in patients with moderate to severe OSA. Sleep 2011;34(1):111–9.

24. Walia HK, Griffith SD, Foldvary-Schaefer N, et al. Longitudinal effect of CPAP on BP in resistant and nonresistant hypertension in a large clinic-based Cohort. Chest 2016;149(3):747–55.

25. Law MR, Morris JK, Wald NJ. Use of blood pressure lowering drugs in the prevention of cardiovascular disease: meta-analysis of 147 randomised trials in the context of expectations from prospective epidemiological studies. BMJ 2009;338:b1665.

26. Sin DD, Mayers I, Man GC, et al. Long-term compliance rates to continuous positive airway pressure in obstructive sleep apnea: a population-based study. Chest 2002;121(2):430–5.

27. Budhiraja R, Parthasarathy S, Drake CL, et al. Early CPAP use identifies subsequent adherence to CPAP therapy. Sleep 2007;30(3):320–4.

28. Pieters T, Collard P, Aubert G, et al. Acceptance and long-term compliance with nCPAP in patients with obstructive sleep apnoea syndrome. Eur Respir J 1996;9(5):939–44.

29. Billings ME, Auckley D, Benca R, et al. Race and residential socioeconomics as predictors of CPAP adherence. Sleep 2011;34(12):1653–8.

30. Campbell A, Neill A, Lory R. Ethnicity and socioeconomic status predict initial continuous positive airway pressure compliance in New Zealand adults with obstructive sleep apnoea. Intern Med J 2012;42(6):e95–101.

31. Platt AB, Field SH, Asch DA, et al. Neighborhood of residence is associated with daily adherence to CPAP therapy. Sleep 2009;32(6):799–806.

32. Scharf SM, Seiden L, DeMore J, et al. Racial differences in clinical presentation of patients with sleep-disordered breathing. Sleep Breath 2004;8(4):173–83.

33. Loube DI, Gay PC, Strohl KP, et al. Indications for positive airway pressure treatment of adult obstructive sleep apnea patients: a consensus statement. Chest 1999;115(3):863–6.

34. Li HY, Engleman H, Hsu CY, et al. Acoustic reflection for nasal airway measurement in patients with obstructive sleep apnea-hypopnea syndrome. Sleep 2005;28(12):1554–9.

35. Morris LG, Setlur J, Burschtin OE, et al. Acoustic rhinometry predicts tolerance of nasal continuous positive airway pressure: a pilot study. Am J Rhinol 2006;20(2):133–7.

36. Wickwire EM, Lettieri CJ, Cairns AA, et al. Maximizing positive airway pressure adherence in adults: a common-sense approach. Chest 2013;144(2):680–93.

37. Dzierzewski JM, Wallace DM, Wohlgemuth WK. Adherence to continuous positive airway pressure in existing users: self-efficacy enhances the association between continuous positive airway

pressure and adherence. J Clin Sleep Med 2016; 12(2):169–76.

38. Aloia MS, Arnedt JT, Stanchina M, et al. How early in treatment is PAP adherence established? Revisiting night-to-night variability. Behav Sleep Med 2007;5(3):229–40.

39. Lewis KE, Seale L, Bartle IE, et al. Early predictors of CPAP use for the treatment of obstructive sleep apnea. Sleep 2004;27(1):134–8.

40. Drake CL, Day R, Hudgel D, et al. Sleep during titration predicts continuous positive airway pressure compliance. Sleep 2003;26(3):308–11.

41. Balachandran JS, Yu X, Wroblewski K, et al. A brief survey of patients' first impression after CPAP titration predicts future CPAP adherence: a pilot study. J Clin Sleep Med 2013;9(3):199–205.

42. Poulet C, Veale D, Arnol N, et al. Psychological variables as predictors of adherence to treatment by continuous positive airway pressure. Sleep Med 2009;10(9):993–9.

43. Sawyer AM, King TS, Sawyer DA, et al. Is inconsistent pre-treatment bedtime related to CPAP non-adherence? Res Nurs Health 2014;37(6):504–11.

44. Russo-Magno P, O'Brien A, Panciera T, et al. Compliance with CPAP therapy in older men with obstructive sleep apnea. J Am Geriatr Soc 2001; 49(9):1205–11.

45. Woehrle H, Graml A, Weinreich G. Age- and gender-dependent adherence with continuous positive airway pressure therapy. Sleep Med 2011;12(10):1034–6.

46. Walter RJ, Lettieri CJ, Sheikh K, et al. Does medication adherence predict cpap compliance? Sleep 2015;36:A200.

47. Engleman HM, Wild MR. Improving CPAP use by patients with the sleep apnoea/hypopnoea syndrome (SAHS). Sleep Med Rev 2003;7(1):81–99.

48. Borel JC, Tamisier R, Dias-Domingos S, et al. Type of mask may impact on continuous positive airway pressure adherence in apneic patients. PLoS One 2013;8(5):e64382.

49. Anderson FE, Kingshott RN, Taylor DR, et al. A randomized crossover efficacy trial of oral CPAP (Oracle) compared with nasal CPAP in the management of obstructive sleep apnea. Sleep 2003; 26(6):721–6.

50. Beecroft J, Zanon S, Lukic D, et al. Oral continuous positive airway pressure for sleep apnea: effectiveness, patient preference, and adherence. Chest 2003;124(6):2200–8.

51. Khanna R, Kline LR. A prospective 8 week trial of nasal interfaces vs. a novel oral interface (Oracle) for treatment of obstructive sleep apnea hypopnea syndrome. Sleep Med 2003;4(4):333–8.

52. Mortimore IL, Whittle AT, Douglas NJ. Comparison of nose and face mask CPAP therapy for sleep apnoea. Thorax 1998;53(4):290–2.

53. Ryan S, Garvey JF, Swan V, et al. Nasal pillows as an alternative interface in patients with obstructive sleep apnoea syndrome initiating continuous positive airway pressure therapy. J Sleep Res 2011; 20(2):367–73.

54. Schorr F, Genta PR, Gregorio MG, et al. Continuous positive airway pressure delivered by oronasal mask may not be effective for obstructive sleep apnoea. Eur Respir J 2012;40(2):503–5.

55. Bachour A, Vitikainen P, Maasilta P. Rates of initial acceptance of PAP masks and outcomes of mask switching. Sleep Breath 2016;20(2):733–8.

56. Bachour A, Vitikainen P, Virkkula P, et al. CPAP interface: satisfaction and side effects. Sleep Breath 2013;17(2):667–72.

57. Deshpande S, Joosten S, Turton A, et al. Oronasal masks require a higher pressure than nasal and nasal pillow masks for the treatment of obstructive sleep apnea. J Clin Sleep Med 2016;12(9):1263–8.

58. Ebben MR, Narizhnaya M, Segal AZ, et al. A randomised controlled trial on the effect of mask choice on residual respiratory events with continuous positive airway pressure treatment. Sleep Med 2014; 15(6):619–24.

59. Ng JR, Aiyappan V, Mercer J, et al. Choosing an oronasal mask to deliver continuous positive airway pressure may cause more upper airway obstruction or lead to higher continuous positive airway pressure requirements than a nasal mask in some patients: a case series. J Clin Sleep Med 2016; 12(9):1227–32.

60. Kaliner MA, Osguthorpe JD, Fireman P, et al. Sinusitis: bench to bedside. Current findings, future directions. J Allergy Clin Immunol 1997;99(6 Pt 3): S829–48.

61. Ulander M, Johansson MS, Ewaldh AE, et al. Side effects to continuous positive airway pressure treatment for obstructive sleep apnoea: changes over time and association to adherence. Sleep Breath 2014;18(4):799–807.

62. Alahmari MD, Sapsford RJ, Wedzicha JA, et al. Dose response of continuous positive airway pressure on nasal symptoms, obstruction and inflammation in vivo and in vitro. Eur Respir J 2012; 40(5):1180–90.

63. Koutsourelakis I, Vagiakis E, Perraki E, et al. Nasal inflammation in sleep apnoea patients using CPAP and effect of heated humidification. Eur Respir J 2011;37(3):587–94.

64. Beneto A, Gomez-Siurana E, Rubio-Sanchez P. Comorbidity between sleep apnea and insomnia. Sleep Med Rev 2009;13(4):287–93.

65. Krakow B, Melendrez D, Ferreira E, et al. Prevalence of insomnia symptoms in patients with sleep-disordered breathing. Chest 2001;120(6): 1923–9.

66. Krakow B, Melendrez D, Lee SA, et al. Refractory insomnia and sleep-disordered breathing: a pilot study. Sleep Breath 2004;8(1):15–29.

67. Krakow B, Melendrez D, Warner TD, et al. To breathe, perchance to sleep: sleep-disordered breathing and chronic insomnia among trauma survivors. Sleep Breath 2002;6(4):189–202.

68. Wickwire EM, Smith MT, Birnbaum S, et al. Sleep maintenance insomnia complaints predict poor CPAP adherence: a clinical case series. Sleep Med 2010;11(8):772–6.

69. Collen JF, Lettieri CJ, Hoffman M. The impact of posttraumatic stress disorder on CPAP adherence in patients with obstructive sleep apnea. J Clin Sleep Med 2012;8(6):667–72.

70. El-Solh AA, Ayyar L, Akinnusi M, et al. Positive airway pressure adherence in veterans with posttraumatic stress disorder. Sleep 2010;33(11): 1495–500.

71. Lettieri CJ, Williams SG, Collen JF. OSA syndrome and posttraumatic stress disorder: clinical outcomes and impact of positive airway pressure therapy. Chest 2016;149(2):483–90.

72. Lettieri CJ, Shah AA, Holley AB, et al. Effects of a short course of eszopiclone on continuous positive airway pressure adherence: a randomized trial. Ann Intern Med 2009;151(10): 696–702.

73. National Institute of Health, et al. NIH Consens State Sci Statements 2005;22:1.

74. Qaseem A, Kansagara D, Forciea MA, et al, Clinical Guidelines Committee of the American College of Physicians. Management of chronic insomnia disorder in adults: a clinical practice guideline from the American College of Physicians. Ann Intern Med 2016;165(2):125–33.

75. Schutte-Rodin S, Broch L, Buysse D, et al. Clinical guideline for the evaluation and management of chronic insomnia in adults. J Clin Sleep Med 2008;4(5):487–504.

76. Luyster FS, Buysse DJ, Strollo PJ Jr. Comorbid insomnia and obstructive sleep apnea: challenges for clinical practice and research. J Clin Sleep Med 2010;6(2):196–204.

77. Chasens ER, Pack AI, Maislin G, et al. Claustrophobia and adherence to CPAP treatment. West J Nurs Res 2005;27(3):307–21.

78. Haynes PL. The role of behavioral sleep medicine in the assessment and treatment of sleep disordered breathing. Clin Psychol Rev 2005;25(5): 673–705.

79. Krakow B, Ulibarri V, Melendrez D, et al. A daytime, abbreviated cardio-respiratory sleep study (CPT 95807-52) to acclimate insomnia patients with sleep disordered breathing to positive airway pressure (PAP-NAP). J Clin Sleep Med 2008;4(3): 212–22.

80. Jurado-Gamez B, Bardwell WA, Cordova-Pacheco LJ, et al. A basic intervention improves CPAP adherence in sleep apnoea patients: a controlled trial. Sleep Breath 2015;19(2):509–14.

81. Basoglu OK, Midilli M, Midilli R, et al. Adherence to continuous positive airway pressure therapy in obstructive sleep apnea syndrome: effect of visual education. Sleep Breath 2012;16(4): 1193–200.

82. Jean Wiese H, Boethel C, Phillips B, et al. CPAP compliance: video education may help! Sleep Med 2005;6(2):171–4.

83. Chervin RD, Theut S, Bassetti C, et al. Compliance with nasal CPAP can be improved by simple interventions. Sleep 1997;20(4):284–9.

84. Brostrom A, Fridlund B, Ulander M, et al. A mixed method evaluation of a group-based educational programme for CPAP use in patients with obstructive sleep apnea. J Eval Clin Pract 2013;19(1): 173–84.

85. Aloia MS, Di Dio L, Ilniczky N, et al. Improving compliance with nasal CPAP and vigilance in older adults with OAHS. Sleep Breath 2001;5(1): 13–21.

86. Sedkaoui K, Leseux L, Pontier S, et al. Efficiency of a phone coaching program on adherence to continuous positive airway pressure in sleep apnea hypopnea syndrome: a randomized trial. BMC Pulm Med 2015;15:102.

87. Aloia MS, Arnedt JT, Riggs RL, et al. Clinical management of poor adherence to CPAP: motivational enhancement. Behav Sleep Med 2004;2(4): 205–22.

88. Bartlett D, Wong K, Richards D, et al. Increasing adherence to obstructive sleep apnea treatment with a group social cognitive therapy treatment intervention: a randomized trial. Sleep 2013; 36(11):1647–54.

89. Edinger JD, Radtke RA. Use of in vivo desensitization to treat a patient's claustrophobic response to nasal CPAP. Sleep 1993;16(7):678–80.

90. Lai AY, Fong DY, Lam JC, et al. The efficacy of a brief motivational enhancement education program on CPAP adherence in OSA: a randomized controlled trial. Chest 2014;146(3):600–10.

91. Olsen S, Smith SS, Oei TP, et al. Motivational interviewing (MINT) improves continuous positive airway pressure (CPAP) acceptance and adherence: a randomized controlled trial. J Consult Clin Psychol 2012;80(1):151–63.

92. Richards D, Bartlett DJ, Wong K, et al. Increased adherence to CPAP with a group cognitive behavioral treatment intervention: a randomized trial. Sleep 2007;30(5):635–40.

93. Ye L, Malhotra A, Kayser K, et al. Spousal involvement and CPAP adherence: a dyadic perspective. Sleep Med Rev 2015;19:67–74.

94. Wozniak DR, Lasserson TJ, Smith I. Educational, supportive and behavioural interventions to improve usage of continuous positive airway pressure machines in adults with obstructive sleep apnoea. Cochrane Database Syst Rev 2014;(1): CD007736.

95. Weaver TE, Maislin G, Dinges DF, et al. Self-efficacy in sleep apnea: instrument development and patient perceptions of obstructive sleep apnea risk, treatment benefit, and volition to use continuous positive airway pressure. Sleep 2003;26(6): 727–32.

96. McArdle N, Kingshott R, Engleman HM, et al. Partners of patients with sleep apnoea/hypopnoea syndrome: effect of CPAP treatment on sleep quality and quality of life. Thorax 2001;56(7): 513–8.

97. Cartwright R. Sleeping together: a pilot study of the effects of shared sleeping on adherence to CPAP treatment in obstructive sleep apnea. J Clin Sleep Med 2008;4(2):123–7.

98. Doherty LS, Kiely JL, Lawless G, et al. Impact of nasal continuous positive airway pressure therapy on the quality of life of bed partners of patients with obstructive sleep apnea syndrome. Chest 2003;124(6):2209–14.

99. McFadyen TA, Espie CA, McArdle N, et al. Controlled, prospective trial of psychosocial function before and after continuous positive airway pressure therapy. Eur Respir J 2001;18(6): 996–1002.

100. Parish JM, Lyng PJ. Quality of life in bed partners of patients with obstructive sleep apnea or hypopnea after treatment with continuous positive airway pressure. Chest 2003;124(3):942–7.

101. Lettieri CJ, Walter RJ. Impact of group education on continuous positive airway pressure adherence. J Clin Sleep Med 2013;9(6):537–41.

102. Miller WR, Rollnick S. Motivational interviewing: helping people change. 3rd edition. New York: Guilford Press; 2013.

103. Aloia MS, Smith K, Arnedt JT, et al. Brief behavioral therapies reduce early positive airway pressure discontinuation rates in sleep apnea syndrome: preliminary findings. Behav Sleep Med 2007;5(2): 89–104.

104. Bakker JP, Wang R, Weng J, et al. Motivational enhancement for increasing adherence to CPAP: a randomized controlled trial. Chest 2016;150(2): 337–45.

105. Dantas AP, Winck JC, Figueiredo-Braga M. Adherence to APAP in obstructive sleep apnea syndrome: effectiveness of a motivational intervention. Sleep Breath 2015;19(1):327–34.

106. Schwab RJ, Badr SM, Epstein LJ, et al. An official American Thoracic Society statement: continuous positive airway pressure adherence tracking systems. The optimal monitoring strategies and outcome measures in adults. Am J Respir Crit Care Med 2013;188(5):613–20.

107. Haniffa M, Lasserson TJ, Smith I. Interventions to improve compliance with continuous positive airway pressure for obstructive sleep apnoea. Cochrane Database Syst Rev 2004;(4):CD003531.

108. Massie CA, Hart RW, Peralez K, et al. Effects of humidification on nasal symptoms and compliance in sleep apnea patients using continuous positive airway pressure. Chest 1999;116(2):403–8.

109. Aloia MS, Stanchina M, Arnedt JT, et al. Treatment adherence and outcomes in flexible vs standard continuous positive airway pressure therapy. Chest 2005;127(6):2085–93.

110. Chihara Y, Tsuboi T, Hitomi T, et al. Flexible positive airway pressure improves treatment adherence compared with auto-adjusting PAP. Sleep 2013; 36(2):229–36.

111. Berry RB, Patel PB. Effect of zolpidem on the efficacy of continuous positive airway pressure as treatment for obstructive sleep apnea. Sleep 2006;29(8):1052–6.

112. Bradshaw DA, Ruff GA, Murphy DP. An oral hypnotic medication does not improve continuous positive airway pressure compliance in men with obstructive sleep apnea. Chest 2006;130(5): 1369–76.

113. Coyle MA, Mendelson WB, Derchak PA, et al. Ventilatory safety of zaleplon during sleep in patients with obstructive sleep apnea on continuous positive airway pressure. J Clin Sleep Med 2005; 1(1):97.

114. Collen J, Lettieri C, Kelly W, et al. Clinical and polysomnographic predictors of short-term continuous positive airway pressure compliance. Chest 2009; 135(3):704–9.

115. Lettieri CJ, Collen JF, Eliasson AH, et al. Sedative use during continuous positive airway pressure titration improves subsequent compliance: a randomized, double-blind, placebo-controlled trial. Chest 2009;136(5):1263–8.

116. Lettieri CJ, Eliasson AH, Andrada T, et al. Does zolpidem enhance the yield of polysomnography? J Clin Sleep Med 2005;1(2):129–31.

117. Lettieri CJ, Quast TN, Eliasson AH, et al. Eszopiclone improves overnight polysomnography and continuous positive airway pressure titration: a prospective, randomized, placebo-controlled trial. Sleep 2008;31(9):1310–6.

118. Zhang XJ, Li QY, Wang Y, et al. The effect of non-benzodiazepine hypnotics on sleep quality and severity in patients with OSA: a meta-analysis. Sleep Breath 2014;18(4):781–9.

119. Eckert DJ, Owens RL, Kehlmann GB, et al. Eszopiclone increases the respiratory arousal threshold and lowers the apnoea/hypopnoea index in

obstructive sleep apnoea patients with a low arousal threshold. Clin Sci (Lond) 2011;120(12):505–14.

120. Edwards BA, Eckert DJ, McSharry DG, et al. Clinical predictors of the respiratory arousal threshold in patients with obstructive sleep apnea. Am J Respir Crit Care Med 2014;190(11):1293–300.

121. Shepherd K, Hillman D, Eastwood P. CPAP-induced aerophagia may precipitate gastroesophageal reflux. J Clin Sleep Med 2013;9(6):633–4.

122. Shepherd K, Hillman D, Eastwood P. Symptoms of aerophagia are common in patients on continuous positive airway pressure therapy and are related to the presence of nighttime gastroesophageal reflux. J Clin Sleep Med 2013;9(1):13–7.

123. Watson NF, Mystkowski SK. Aerophagia and gastroesophageal reflux disease in patients using continuous positive airway pressure: a preliminary observation. J Clin Sleep Med 2008; 4(5):434–8.

124. Morgenthaler TI, Kuzniar TJ, Wolfe LF, et al. The complex sleep apnea resolution study: a prospective randomized controlled trial of continuous positive airway pressure versus adaptive

servoventilation therapy. Sleep 2014;37(5): 927–34.

125. Kuzniar TJ, Morgenthaler TI. Treatment of complex sleep apnea syndrome. Chest 2012;142(4): 1049–57.

126. Dellweg D, Kerl J, Hoehn E, et al. Randomized controlled trial of noninvasive positive pressure ventilation (NPPV) versus servoventilation in patients with CPAP-induced central sleep apnea (complex sleep apnea). Sleep 2013;36(8): 1163–71.

127. Cowie MR, Woehrle H, Wegscheider K, et al. Adaptive servo-ventilation for central sleep apnea in systolic heart failure. N Engl J Med 2015;373(12): 1095–105.

128. Yamaguti WP, Moderno EV, Yamashita SY, et al. Treatment-related risk factors for development of skin breakdown in subjects with acute respiratory failure undergoing noninvasive ventilation or CPAP. Respir Care 2014;59(10):1530–6.

129. Tsuda H, Almeida FR, Tsuda T, et al. Craniofacial changes after 2 years of nasal continuous positive airway pressure use in patients with obstructive sleep apnea. Chest 2010;138:870–4.

# Positive Airway Pressure Therapy for Hyperventilatory Central Sleep Apnea

## Idiopathic, Heart Failure, Cerebrovascular Disease, and High Altitude

Shahrokh Javaheri, MD[a,b,c],*, Lee K. Brown, MD[d,e]

## KEYWORDS

- Central sleep apnea • Hunter-Cheyne-Stokes breathing • Heart failure • High altitude
- Cerebrovascular disease • Adaptive servoventilation • Bilevel positive airway pressure
- Continuous positive airway pressure

## KEY POINTS

- Hyperventilatory central sleep apnea (CSA) and Hunter-Cheyne-Stokes breathing (HCSB) are caused by a temporary failure in the pontomedullary pacemaker generating breathing rhythm, caused by the existence of an apneic threshold for arterial $P_{CO_2}$ confined primarily to non–rapid eye movement sleep.
- Common causes of hyperventilatory CSA/HCSB in adults are congestive heart failure and stroke.
- Diagnosis and treatment of hyperventilatory CSA/HCSB may improve quality of life, and, when associated with heart failure or cerebrovascular disease, reduce morbidity and perhaps mortality.
- Treatment choices for hyperventilatory CSA/HCSB may include exogenous oxygen administration; continuous positive airway pressure; bilevel positive airway pressure (usually with a backup rate); and, more recently, adaptive servoventilation. Another treatment, phrenic nerve stimulation, is currently under investigation but is beyond of the scope of this article.

Financial Disclosures: S. Javaheri has no relevant conflicts of interest. L.K. Brown has participated in advisory panels for Philips Respironics, and is an insurance claims reviewer for Considine and Associates, Inc. He coedits the sleep and respiratory neurobiology section of *Current Opinion in Pulmonary Medicine*, wrote on continuous positive airway pressure treatment of obstructive sleep apnea in UpToDate and on obstructive sleep apnea in Clinical Decision Support: Pulmonary Medicine and Sleep Disorders. He is currently coediting an issue of *Sleep Medicine Clinics* on positive airway pressure therapy. He serves on the Polysomnography Practice Advisory Committee of the New Mexico Medical Board and chairs the New Mexico Respiratory Care Advisory Board.

[a] Sleep Laboratory, Bethesda North Hospital, 10535 Montgomery Road, Suite 200, Cincinnati, OH 45242, USA;
[b] The University of Cincinnati, Cincinnati, OH, USA; [c] The Ohio University Medical School, Columbus, OH, USA;
[d] Division of Pulmonary, Critical Care, and Sleep Medicine, Department of Internal Medicine, University of New Mexico School of Medicine, University of New Mexico Sleep Disorders Center, 1101 Medical Arts Avenue Northeast, Building #2, Albuquerque, NM 87102, USA; [e] Department of Electrical and Computer Engineering, University of New Mexico School of Engineering, University of New Mexico Sleep Disorders Center, 1101 Medical Arts Avenue Northeast, Building #2, Albuquerque, NM 87102, USA
* Corresponding author. Bethesda North Hospital, 10535 Montgomery Road, Suite 200, Cincinnati, OH 45242.
E-mail address: shahrokhjavaheri@icloud.com

Sleep Med Clin 12 (2017) 565–572
http://dx.doi.org/10.1016/j.jsmc.2017.07.006
1556-407X/17/© 2017 Elsevier Inc. All rights reserved.

# INTRODUCTION

Central sleep apnea (CSA) and its variant Hunter-Cheyne-Stokes breathing (HCSB) result when respiratory rhythmogenesis temporarily fails to initiate inspiration or, in the case of HCSB, rhythmogenesis is aberrant in that there is a waning and waxing of inspiratory effort separated by a (usually brief) period of central apnea. This discordant breathing could be the result of varied medical conditions, although even in normal individuals a few central apneas may be observed during polysomnography in the absence of any pathologic condition (physiologic central apnea), particularly on the resumption of sleep; after an arousal or awakening.[1] One important group of disorders causing CSA/HCSB is characterized by the presence of diurnal hyperventilation, or low normal values for arterial $P_{CO_2}$, and positive airway pressure (PAP) treatment of these disorders is the focus of this article. A comprehensive list of causes of CSA/HCSB, the underlying mechanisms, and other therapeutic options are beyond the scope of this article and have been covered previously.[1–5]

# IDIOPATHIC CENTRAL SLEEP APNEA

This is a rare polysomnographic finding in individuals otherwise thought to be free of comorbidities. There are multiple causes of CSA in otherwise asymptomatic individuals and some may have unrecognized disorders that might be the cause of the so-called idiopathic CSA. Examples include asymptomatic carotid artery stenosis and left ventricular systolic dysfunction. These potential causes of CSA, and others, were not systematically investigated in most reports of idiopathic CSA. Therefore, before any specific therapy for CSA with PAP devices or with pharmacologic therapy is contemplated, appropriate testing for a potential cause should be undertaken and, if found, appropriately treated. For example, surgical treatment of carotid artery stenosis may be all that is needed to eliminate what was considered idiopathic CSA. The HCSB variant of CSA has occasionally been reported to be idiopathic, but it is likely that one of the underlying causes mentioned earlier could have been present but not identified.

There are no systematic studies on PAP therapy in idiopathic CSA. If no cause is found, the authors recommend a trial of continuous PAP (CPAP) as the first treatment modality. If ineffective, we recommend pharmacologic therapy. Bilevel PAP devices in spontaneous mode (bilevel PAP-S) should not be used to treat CSA whatever the underlying disorder, because these devices could result in worsening of central apnea by increasing ventilation, reducing the prevailing arterial $P_{CO_2}$ below the apneic threshold for $P_{CO_2}$, and creating a vicious cycle of worsening CSA.[6] This phenomenon was reported in a patient with idiopathic CSA treated with bilevel PAP-S.[7] If bilevel PAP is used, a backup rate (timed mode) should always be used (bilevel PAP-S/T). However, the new generation of adaptive servoventilators (ASVs)[8] should in theory be most effective and comfortable but no data exist specifically for this modality in patients with truly idiopathic CSA.

# HEART FAILURE

Sleep disordered breathing (SDB), both obstructive and CSA/HCSB, commonly occurs in individuals with left ventricular dysfunction, which may be both systolic and diastolic. Most commonly CSA/HCSB occurs in patients with heart failure with reduced ejection fraction (HFrEF) and those with heart failure with preserved ejection fraction (HFpEF). However, CSA/HCSB caused by left ventricular dysfunction often manifests the unique pattern of periodic breathing described as HCSB.[2] The pattern of HCSB is characterized by central apneas that occur between decrescendo-crescendo ventilatory efforts. Importantly, as in the case of obstructive sleep apnea (OSA), central apneas also result in hypoxia alternating with reoxygenation, changes in arterial $P_{CO_2}$, and recurrent arousals. Furthermore, central apneas are associated with excessive negative swings in intrathoracic pressure during the hyperventilatory phase of the cycle, also bearing similarity to those that occur in OSA. These adverse consequences of CSA/HCSB are generally of a lesser degree compared with those accompanying OSA. However, multiple studies have shown that, compared with patients with heart failure without central sleep apnea, those with CSA do have adverse consequences, most likely caused by the creation of a hyperadrenergic state. This hyperadrenergic state has been shown using a variety of techniques, including muscle sympathetic nerve activity, plasma and urinary norepinephrine measurements, and heart rate variability. In addition, multiple randomized clinical trials, mostly incorporating small numbers of patients, have shown that attenuation of CSA/HCSB by PAP therapy, including CPAP and ASV, as well as by nocturnal oxygen administration, attenuates the hyperadrenergic state imposed by central SDB.[3] This article reviews the studies with CPAP and adaptive servoventilation; the authors do not recommend the use of bilevel PAP-S for CSA, as noted earlier. Virtually all studies using a PAP device, specifically CPAP and ASV, have shown beneficial effects on various outcomes in patients with heart failure and CSA. The exception is a recent phase 3 randomized controlled trial using a previous-generation ASV device in patients with HFrEF, which not only failed to show any improvement in either hospitalization or all-cause mortality but, in contradiction, purportedly showed an increase in cardiovascular mortality.[9]

In 1990, the authors reported the successful use of CPAP to treat a patient with CSA/HCSB with HFrEF.[10] We were initially planning to treat the patient with theophylline, but the patient indicated a preference for attempting nondrug therapy first. More systematic studies of CPAP for CSA/HCSB in heart failure followed; in one study of the acute effects, overnight CSA/HCSB was eliminated in about 40% of the patients with heart failure.[11] Importantly, ventricular arrhythmias were acutely suppressed by the use of CPAP only in those patients whose CSA/HCSB was suppressed by CPAP. Multiple studies from the Toronto group show that attenuation of CSA/HCSB by CPAP results in a reduction in plasma and urinary catecholamine levels and improved ejection fraction within months of nightly treatment. These short-term studies were followed by the Canadian Continuous Positive Airway Pressure for Patients with Central Sleep Apnea and Heart Failure (CANPAP) trial, the only randomized long-term (2 years) controlled multicenter trial of CPAP therapy in patients with HFrEF and CSA/HCSB. Surprisingly, this trial did not show improved overall transplant-free survival of patients with HFrEF on treatment.[12] In an editorial based on our previous experience noted earlier, we predicted that the reason for the overall neutral result was the presence of a subgroup of patients with heart failure in whom CPAP had failed to improve their CSA/HCSB.[13] In all of the treated patients, the increased intrathoracic pressure imposed by CPAP could adversely affect preload and afterload and impair hemodynamics. However, in those patients in whom CPAP successfully suppressed CSA/HCSB, the benefits thereby derived could have outweighed the adverse hemodynamic effects, resulting in a neutral outcome. Pump failure and sudden death were the most common causes of death or adverse outcome in both the control arm and the CPAP arm, and these are the 2 most common causes of demise in patients with heart failure.

In the CANPAP trial, patients were brought to the hospital and were titrated with CPAP starting from a pressure of 5 cm $H_2O$ to a maximum of 10 to 12 cm $H_2O$ during an overnight observation. The patients were discharged for home treatment at the maximum tolerable CPAP level. Patients were brought back to the sleep laboratory at 3 months and, for the first time, had nocturnal polysomnography on their CPAP to determine responsiveness. This testing identified 2 subgroups: a cohort of patients in whom CPAP effectively suppressed their CSA/HCSB and a cohort of patients who were unresponsive to CPAP. In those in whom CSA/HCSB was suppressed, the mean apnea-hypopnea index (AHI) decreased from a mean baseline value of about 40 per hour of sleep to a mean of 6 per hour of sleep. In those in whom CPAP failed to suppress CSA, the mean AHI decreased from about 40 per hour of sleep to 36 per hour of sleep at 3 months, which was clearly an insignificant change. A post hoc analysis of mortality comparing the two subgroups confirmed significantly improved survival time of CPAP responders compared with CPAP nonresponders and the control group.[14] It also seemed that survival of the CPAP nonresponders was inferior to that of the control group, although the latter finding was not significant given the small number of patients. It should be emphasized that these are post hoc analyses and hold less weight than the primary outcome analysis for which the trial was designed. Other weaknesses of the CANPAP trial have also been identified, including the low numbers of enrollees compared with what was planned, as well as radical changes in guideline-based management of heart failure that were taking place during the course of the trial, most significantly the increased use of β-blockers.

The technology and algorithms underlying ASV were developed because almost 40% to 50% of patients with HFrEF and CSA/HCSB do not respond to CPAP.[15] These devices have undergone continuous development, with additional features added as each generation emerged (for more discussion, please see Lee K. Brown and Shahrokh Javaheri's article, "Positive Airway Pressure Device Technology Past and Present: What's in the "Black Box"?," in this issue). In terms of treatment of hyperventilatory CSA/HCSB, the most significant aspect of these devices consists of the anticyclic nature of the degree of inspiratory pressure support, relative to the cyclic pattern of the patient's intrinsic ventilatory drive. The algorithms underlying both of the ASV devices marketed in the United States maintain minimal pressure support during the hyperventilatory phase of CSA/HCSB (when the patient's own ventilatory drive is maximal), and increase pressure support during the hypoventilatory phase when the patient's own ventilatory drive is minimal. Consequently, ASVs dampen the fluctuations in arterial $P_{CO_2}$ which, by interacting with peripheral and central chemoreceptors, promotes the unstable periodic breathing pattern exemplified by CSA/HCSB. As expected, studies using ASV devices in patients with heart failure showed superior efficacy in eliminating CSA/HCSB compared with other modalities, and in turn a consistent finding of reduced sympathetic tone and improved ejection fraction.[3,8] A meta-analysis published by the authors in 2012 reviewed available data of studies involving patients with heart failure in which ASV treatment was compared with therapy with either oxygen, CPAP, bilevel PAP, or standard of care.[16] We unequivocally showed that ASV was the most effective treatment modality and was associated with consistent improvements in ejection fraction. Given the wealth of literature supporting the use of ASV in both HFrEF and HFpEF in terms of surrogate or intermediate end points, the release of the adverse findings of the Treatment of Sleep-Disordered Breathing with Predominant Central Sleep Apnea by Adaptive Servo Ventilation in Patients with Heart Failure (SERVE-HF) trial took the medical community by surprise.[9]

The SERVE-HF study was a multicenter randomized controlled trial designed to compare the effect of standard guideline-based medical management plus ASV versus medical management alone in 1325 patients with chronic HFrEF, defined as a left ventricular ejection fraction less than or equal to 45%. Patients enrolled had an AHI greater than or equal to 15 events per hour with CSA/HCSB predominating. There was no statistically significant difference in the primary end point, which was a composite of first event of death from any cause, lifesaving cardiovascular intervention, or unplanned hospitalization for worsening heart failure (hazard ratio = 1.14; 95% confidence interval, 0.97–1.33; $P$ = .10). Thus, in terms of the primary end point that drove the statistical design of the study, the results were neutral, the same as in the CANPAP trial.[12] However, an analysis of secondary end points revealed a statistically significant increased risk of cardiovascular mortality with ASV compared with control. However, with regard to survival, there were important differences between the CANPAP and SERVE-HF trials. In the CANPAP trial, excess mortality in the CPAP arm occurred early on but, over time, survival favored CPAP, although by the end of the study there was still no significant difference overall.[12] In contrast, the SERVE-HF trial found a progressive annual increase of 2.5% in mortality with ASV compared with guideline-based therapy alone.

The investigators of the SERVE-HF report speculated that, given the significant improvement in AHI experienced by the patients in the ASV arm, CSA/HCSB might represent a compensatory, protective, and adaptive mechanism in HFrEF that could enhance survival,[9] a theory that had been previously advanced by Naughton.[17] In other words, CSA in HFrEF need not be treated. However, as reviewed in detail elsewhere, there were multiple defects in the design, management, and analysis of SERVE-HF that could explain the adverse findings that were reported.[18] An important strategic issue was the use of the first generation of ASV technology (no longer marketed in the United States), which may have doomed the study to failure. These problems have been resolved in the new-generation ASV devices.[8,15] As an example, sleep apnea in patients with HFrEF frequently manifests as a mixture of central and obstructive events, and the phenotype in many patients is known to change across the night and over the course of days, weeks, and months. In SERVE-HF, even though 80% of all SDB was considered central in mechanism at the time of enrollment, with time this percentage decreased considerably in favor of more obstructive events. It may be that the ASV technology used was capable of treating central events but not able to effectively control the emergence of obstructive events. This finding was expected, because the ASV device used in SERVE-HF used a fixed level of expiratory PAP (EPAP) and did not incorporate the ability to simultaneously titrate EPAP while also varying pressure support. This potential explanation for the progressive excess in mortality observed in SERVE-HF should be amenable to exploration by identifying subgroups of patients who developed increasing levels of OSA during the course of the study and determining their contribution to the excess cardiovascular mortality. This question and many others needs to be answered in post hoc analyses, as was done by the CANPAP investigators in their trial. In addition, the results are awaited of an ongoing trial, the Effect of ASV on Survival and Hospital Admissions in HF (ADVENT-HF; NCT01128816) in which an advanced ASV device with autotitrating EPAP is being used.[19,20]

## CEREBROVASCULAR DISORDERS

A wide range of central nervous system disorders are associated with CSA, and, in most, the clinical significance remains to be elucidated. Furthermore, arterial blood gas levels have not always been systematically measured and therefore it is not known whether the pathogenesis is similar to what occurs in heart failure. Consequently, inclusion in the category of CSA may not be applicable to many of these disorders. This article concentrates on stroke, which is the most common neurologic reason for hospitalization, resulting in a heavy burden to the economics of health care. There is a known bidirectional relationship between stroke and SDB, inasmuch as OSA is a known risk factor for stroke, and stroke seems to show a causal relationship to OSA as well as CSA/HCSB.

Several studies have reported on the association between stroke and CSA.[21,22] In a meta-analysis incorporating 29 published reports that used a variety of diagnostic techniques (autoCPAP, limited-channel sleep studies, or full polysomnography), 7% of the 2343 patients presenting with hemorrhagic or ischemic stroke, or transient ischemic attacks, were identified as manifesting CSA.[22] This proportion is significant given that CSA is rarely seen in the general population. An area of controversy exists with respect to whether CSA contributes to the poor quality of life, repeated hospitalizations, or mortality in patients following stroke. The authors note that stroke is frequently associated with atherosclerosis of other vascular beds, including coronary artery atherosclerosis and carotid artery stenosis. Concomitant left ventricular systolic and/or diastolic dysfunction and atrial fibrillation are also more common in stroke.[23–25] These comorbidities can be fairly asymptomatic but still be responsible for the development of CSA.

After stroke, the number of central sleep apneas decreases with time,[26] unless the cause of CSA is another condition, such as atrial fibrillation or heart failure. Moreover, little is known with respect to the mechanisms responsible for the reduction in CSA prevalence with time. Some investigators have reported associations between damage to specific cortical areas and the development of CSA/HCSB: Hermann and colleagues[27] reported imaging studies in 3 patients that identified distinct brain lesions involving autonomic (insula) and volitional (supplementary motor cortex, thalamus) regions known to have effects on respiration. Siccoli and colleagues[28] found that stroke severity/extension increased the likelihood of CSA/HCSB, but reported a lower occurrence of CSA in left insular and mesencephalic stroke, concluding that involvement of distinct brain areas with respiratory control functions was responsible for the development of CSA. A recent study by Fisse and colleagues[29] found no association between the presence of SDB after stroke and lesion location, but did not distinguish obstructive from central SDB and therefore added little to this debate. It is likely that, just as there is often improvement over time in nonrespiratory manifestations of cortical stroke, there may be some return of function in these or other cortical regions associated with the development of CSA/HCSB.

Although there is a well-known relationship between the presence of OSA after stroke and functional outcome, surprisingly little has been reported with respect to the presence of CSA in this regard. One small study of SDB and stroke outcome incorporated only 1 patient with CSA.[30] Two recent meta-analyses failed to report any findings with respect to outcomes specific to CSA after stroke,[31,32] although 1 did find an association between disturbed sleep, which might occur in patients with CSA, and adverse outcomes.[32] The SAS CARE prospective outcomes study seems to have been designed to include a subgroup with CSA.[33] However, consulting the ClinicalTrials.gov Web site indicates that data collection has concluded, but the authors could find no report of results after a search of PubMed.[34] However, there is 1 retrospective single-center study, by Brill and colleagues,[35] reporting on 154 patients with poststroke CSA treated with ASV. Fifteen patients had predominantly CSA related to ischemic stroke when first studied at least 1 month following the event. They were mildly hypocapnic (mean nighttime transcutaneous $P_{CO_2}$, $38 \pm 4.7$ mm Hg in 10 subjects; daytime arterial $P_{CO_2}$, $35.4 \pm 2.8$ mm Hg in the other 5 subjects) and had generally severe SDB with AHI (interquartile range) of 54.4 (25, 63.7) per hour by polysomnography or cardiorespiratory polygraphy. These individuals were older (mean age was $62 \pm 9.4$ years) and were mostly mildly (mean body mass index was $31 \pm 5.6$ kg/m$^2$). The investigators noted that the patients did not have congestive heart failure, although not all patients had echocardiography, and cardiovascular risk factors of the 15 patients included coronary heart disease in 4, atrial fibrillation in 2, and hypertension in 10. Thirteen out of the 15 patients were initially treated with continuous (11 out of 15) and 2 with bilevel PAP devices with unsatisfactory control of CSA/HCSB. Adaptive servoventilation significantly improved AHI to 4.7 (0.5, 9.2) per hour at 3 months and 6.6 (1.5, 11.9) per hour at 6 months (data derived from the device download). The adherence to ASV was excellent with mean nightly use of 5 hours at 3 months and 6 hours and 22 minutes at 6 months. However, because of the retrospective nature of the study the investigators were not able to report neurologic outcomes, although there was a dose-response relationship between decline in Epworth Sleepiness Scale score and hours of ASV use. These data provide support for a large randomized controlled prospective study of poststroke patients with predominantly CSA or combinations of CSA and OSA, using the new generation of ASV devices that are effective in the treatment of both OSA and CSA.

## HIGH ALTITUDE

On sojourn to high altitude, here defined as at or above 2500 to 3000 m, periodic breathing with CSA occurs almost universally. In general, the severity of CSA increases with altitude once a threshold of 2000 m is reached.[4,36]

Individuals who abruptly move to high altitude frequently report sleep disturbances, including insomnia and restlessness. Much of this can be attributed to CSA, which fragments sleep because of arousals, as well as the effects of hypoxia by itself, hypocapnia induced by hypoxia, and concomitant changes in cerebral blood flow. These phenomena collectively result in daytime fatigue and cognitive impairment.[37] The underlying mechanism for CSA is altitude-related hypoxic stimulation of the peripheral chemoreceptors, which reduces arterial $Pco_2$ to below the apneic threshold. This process primarily occurs during non–rapid eye movement (NREM) sleep, because the $Pco_2$ reserve is narrower in NREM sleep than in rapid eye movement sleep and the ventilatory response to arterial $Pco_2$ in NREM is only mildly reduced relative to the more significant reduction during rapid eye movement sleep. Each CSA event results in an increase in arterial $Pco_2$ to above the apneic threshold, ventilation resumes (frequently associated with an arousal), and the cycle repeats throughout NREM sleep.[1,4]

The best pharmacologic treatment of CSA associated with high altitude is prevention by administration of acetazolamide before the sojourn.[4] However, because hypoxia is the fundamental cause of periodic breathing at high altitude, administration of oxygen, when available, is the treatment of choice and readily suppresses CSA.[36]

PAP devices are not always available during most sojourns to high altitude, and only limited information is available on these treatment modalities. Those studies that do exist primarily involve patients with known OSA controlled with CPAP who travel to high altitudes. Such individuals develop CSA and should be warned ahead of time that this can occur.[38–41] Adjunctive treatment with acetazolamide and/or oxygen has been advocated as suitable preventive measures under these circumstances.[40] One recent study suggests that CPAP can ameliorate the effects of altitude on provoking CSA, but this finding has yet to be confirmed; treatment with acetazolamide

and oxygen along with CPAP is still likely to be the best course of action.[42]

Johnson and colleagues[43,44] used CPAP and a bilevel PAP device in separate studies designed to show the effects of these modalities on oxygenation and acute mountain sickness. Both studies suggested a beneficial effect of such treatment, but data on SDB were not reported. These results tended to confirm those of a previous randomized study by Launay and colleagues[45] in which 8 healthy subjects were randomized to positive end-expiratory pressure (PEEP) or no PEEP during acute sojourns to the summit of Mont Blanc (4810 m). Scores for acute mountain sickness were quantified using the Lake Louise acute mountain sickness scoring system. The investigators showed a significant decrease in the incidence and severity of acute mountain sickness with the administration of PEEP, and a trend toward improved oxygenation.

## REFERENCES

1. Javaheri S, Dempsey JA. Central sleep apnea. Compr Physiol 2013;3:141–63.
2. Javaheri S. Heart failure. In: Kryger MH, Roth T, Dement WC, editors. Principles and practices of sleep medicine. 6th edition. Philadelphia: WB Saunders; 2017. p. 1271–85.
3. Brown LK, Javaheri S. Adaptive servoventilation for the treatment of central sleep apnea in congestive heart failure: what have we learned? Curr Opin Pulm Med 2014;20:550–7.
4. Mohsenin V, Javaheri S, Dempsey JA. Sleep and breathing at high altitudes. In: Kryger MH, Roth T, Dement WC, editors. Principles and practices of sleep medicine. 6th edition. Philadelphia: WB Saunders; 2017. p. 1211–21.
5. Randerath WJ, Javaheri S. Adaptive servoventilation in central sleep apnea. Sleep Med Clin 2014;9:69–85.
6. Johnson KG, Johnson DC. Bilevel positive airway pressure worsens central apneas during sleep. Chest 2005;128(4):2141–50.
7. Hommura F, Nishimura M, Oguri M, et al. Continuous versus bilevel positive airway pressure in patients with idiopathic central sleep apnea. Am J Respir Crit Care Med 1997;155:1482–5.
8. Javaheri S, Brown L, Randerath W. Positive airway pressure therapy with adaptive servo-ventilation (part II: clinical applications). Chest 2014;146: 855–68.
9. Cowie MR, Woehrle H, Wegscheider K, et al. Adaptive servo-ventilation for central sleep apnea in systolic heart failure. N Engl J Med 2015;373:1095–105.
10. Dowdell WT, Javaheri S, McGinnis W. Cheyne-Stokes respiration presenting as sleep apnea

syndrome. Clinical and polysomnographic features. Am Rev Respir Dis 1990;141:871–9.

11. Javaheri S, Sands SA, Edwards BA. Acetazolamide attenuates Hunter-Cheyne-Stokes breathing yet paradoxically augments the hypercapnic ventilatory response in patients with heart failure. Ann Am Thorac Soc 2014;11:80–6.

12. Bradley T, Logan A, Kimoff J, et al. Continuous positive airway pressure for central sleep apnea and heart failure. N Engl J Med 2006;353:2025–33.

13. Javaheri S, Shukla R, Zeigler H, et al. Central sleep apnea, right ventricular dysfunction and low diastolic blood pressure are predictors of mortality in systolic heart failure. J Am Coll Cardiol 2007;49:2028–34.

14. Arzt M, Floras JS, Logan AG, et al. Suppression of central sleep apnea by continuous positive airway pressure and transplant-free survival in heart failure. A post-hoc analysis of the Canadian Continuous Positive Airway Pressure for Patients with Central Sleep Apnea and Heart Failure trial (CANPAP). Circulation 2007;115:3173–80.

15. Javaheri S, Brown L, Randerath W. Positive airway pressure therapy with adaptive servoventilation (part 1: operational algorithms). Chest 2014;146: 514–23.

16. Sharma BK, Bakker JP, McSharry DG, et al. Adaptive servoventilation for treatment of sleep-disordered breathing in heart failure: a systematic review and meta-analysis. Chest 2012;142:1211–21.

17. Naughton MT. Cheyne-Stokes respiration: friend or foe? Thorax 2012;67:357–60.

18. Javaheri S, Brown LK, Randerath W, et al. SERVE-HF: more questions than answers [commentary]. Chest 2016;149:900–4.

19. Effect of adaptive servo ventilation (ASV) on survival and hospital admissions in heart failure (ADVENT-HF). Available at: https://clinicaltrials.gov/ct2/show/NCT01128816. Accessed March 12, 2017.

20. Bradley TD, Floras JS, ADVENT-HF Investigators. The SERVE-HF trial. Can Respir J 2015;22:313.

21. Bassetti CL. Sleep and stroke. In: Kryger MH, Roth T, Dement WC, editors. Principles and practices of sleep medicine. 6th edition. Philadelphia: WB Saunders; 2017. p. 903–15.

22. Johnson KG, Johnson DC. Frequency of sleep apnea in stroke and TIA patients: a meta-analysis. J Clin Sleep Med 2010;6:131–7.

23. Nopmaneejumruslers C, Kaneko Y, Hajek V, et al. Cheyne-Stokes respiration in stroke: relationship to hypocapnia and occult cardiac dysfunction. Am J Respir Crit Care Med 2005;171:1048–52.

24. Lavergne F, Morin L, Armitstead J, et al. Atrial fibrillation and sleep-disordered breathing. J Thorac Dis 2015;7:E575–84.

25. Leung RS, Huber MA, Rogge T, et al. Association between atrial fibrillation and central sleep apnea. Sleep 2005;28:1543–6.

26. Parra O, Arboix A, Bechich S, et al. Time course of sleep-related breathing disorders in first-ever stroke or transient ischemic attack. Am J Respir Crit Care Med 2000;161(2 Pt 1):375–80.

27. Hermann DM, Siccoli M, Kirov P, et al. Central periodic breathing during sleep in acute ischemic stroke. Stroke 2007;38:1082–4.

28. Siccoli MM, Valko PO, Hermann DM, et al. Central periodic breathing during sleep in 74 patients with acute ischemic stroke - neurogenic and cardiogenic factors. J Neurol 2008;255:1687–92.

29. Fisse AL, Kemmling A, Teuber A, et al. The association of lesion location and sleep related breathing disorder in patients with acute ischemic stroke. PLoS One 2017;12:e0171243.

30. Yan-fang S, Yu-ping W. Sleep-disordered breathing: impact on functional outcome of ischemic stroke patients. Sleep Med 2009;10:717–9.

31. Birkbak J, Clark AJ, Rod NH. The effect of sleep disordered breathing on the outcome of stroke and transient ischemic attack: a systematic review. J Clin Sleep Med 2014;10:103–8.

32. Hermann DM, Bassetti CL. Role of sleep-disordered breathing and sleep-wake disturbances for stroke and stroke recovery. Neurology 2016;87:1407–16.

33. Cereda CW, Petrini L, Azzola A, et al. Sleep-disordered breathing in acute ischemic stroke and transient ischemic attack: effects on short- and long-term outcome and efficacy of treatment with continuous positive airways pressure–rationale and design of the SAS CARE study. Int J Stroke 2012; 7:597–603.

34. National Institutes of Health. Available at: https://clinicaltrials.gov/ct2/show/NCT01097967. Accessed May 15, 2017.

35. Brill A-K, Rösti R, Hefti JP, et al. Adaptive servo-ventilation as treatment of persistent central sleep apnea in post-acute ischemic stroke patients. Sleep Med 2014;15:1309–13.

36. Burgess KR, Ainslie PN. Central sleep apnea at high altitude. Adv Exp Med Biol 2016;903:275–83.

37. Hota SK, Sharma VK, Hota K, et al. Multi-domain cognitive screening test for neuropsychological assessment for cognitive decline in acclimatized lowlanders staying at high altitude. Indian J Med Res 2012;136:411–20.

38. Bazurto Zapata MA, Martinez-Guzman W, Vargas-Ramirez L, et al. Prevalence of central sleep apnea during continuous positive airway pressure (CPAP) titration in subjects with obstructive sleep apnea syndrome at an altitude of 2640 m. Sleep Med 2015;16:343–6.

39. Nussbaumer-Ochsner Y, Schuepfer N, Ulrich S, et al. Exacerbation of sleep apnoea by frequent central events in patients with the obstructive sleep apnoea syndrome at altitude: a randomised trial. Thorax 2010;65:429–35.

40. Pagel JF, Kwiatkowski C, Parnes B. The effects of altitude associated central apnea on the diagnosis and treatment of obstructive sleep apnea: comparative data from three different altitude locations in the Mountain West. J Clin Sleep Med 2011;7: 610–615A.

41. Latshang TD, Bloch KE. How to treat patients with obstructive sleep apnea syndrome during an altitude sojourn. High Alt Med Biol 2011;12:303–7.

42. Nishida K, Lanspa MJ, Cloward TV, et al. Effects of positive airway pressure on patients with obstructive sleep apnea during acute ascent to altitude. Ann Am Thorac Soc 2015;12:1072–8.

43. Johnson PL, Johnson CC, Poudyal P, et al. Continuous positive airway pressure treatment for acute mountain sickness at 4240 m in the Nepal Himalaya. High Alt Med Biol 2013;14:230–3.

44. Johnson PL, Popa DA, Prisk GK, et al. Non-invasive positive pressure ventilation during sleep at 3800 m: relationship to acute mountain sickness and sleeping oxyhaemoglobin saturation. Respirology 2010;15:277–82.

45. Launay JC, Nespoulos O, Guinet-Lebreton A, et al. Prevention of acute mountain sickness by low positive end-expiratory pressure in field conditions. Scand J Work Environ Health 2004;30:322–6.

# Sleep Disordered Breathing Caused by Chronic Opioid Use
## Diverse Manifestations and Their Management

Susmita Chowdhuri, MD, MS[a],*, Shahrokh Javaheri, MD[b,c,d]

## KEYWORDS

- Central sleep apnea • Obstructive sleep apnea • Ataxic breathing • Biot breathing
- Hypoglossal nerve • Pre-Bötzinger complex • Positive airway pressure • Ampakines

## KEY POINTS

- Obstructive and central apnea and hypopneas, accompanied by cluster and Biot breathing, are common in patients on chronic prescription opioids for noncancer pain. Moreover, sustained hypoxia is noted between respiratory events on polysomnography and hypercapnia is present in a small percentage of patients.
- Opioid-related sleep disordered breathing (SDB) is probably mediated via binding to the pre-Bötzinger complex, hypoglossal nerve nucleus, and chemoreceptor sites.
- Increased hypoxic ventilatory responsiveness, and reduced hypercapnic responsiveness with hypoventilation, may be factors responsible for ventilatory instability during non–rapid eye movement sleep in chronic methadone users.
- Positive airway pressure (PAP)–based therapies offer variable success in eliminating SDB, with adaptive pressure support likely being the most effective. However, long-term outcome data with PAP therapies are not available.
- Ampakine-based therapies are novel agents that counter opioid-induced ventilatory depression without altering their analgesic effect.

## INTRODUCTION

There is an epidemic of prescription opioid use in the United States. Since 1999, sales of prescription opioids have quadrupled.[1] Approximately 11.2% of the adult US population experiences chronic pain[2] and chronic noncancer pain is one of the main reasons for the increase in opioid analgesic use in the United States at a cost of $560 billion to $635 billion annually in medical costs and lost productivity.[3,4] The use of opioid analgesics for pain increased from 3.2% of the population from the period 1988 to 1994 to 5.7% during the period 2005 to 2008.[3] Non–schedule II opioids were the most common

Conflicts of Interest: None.
[a] Sleep Medicine Section, John D. Dingell VA Medical Center, 11 M, 4646 John R Street, Detroit, MI 48201, USA; [b] Medical Director, Montgomery Sleep Laboratory, Cincinnati, OH 45242, USA; [c] University of Cincinnati, College of Medicine, Cincinnati, OH, USA; [d] Division of Cardiology, Department of Internal Medicine, College of Medicine, Ohio State University, Columbus, OH, USA
* Corresponding author.
E-mail address: schowdh@med.wayne.edu

Sleep Med Clin 12 (2017) 573–586
http://dx.doi.org/10.1016/j.jsmc.2017.07.007
1556-407X/17/Published by Elsevier Inc.

type of opioid used in long-term opioid therapy.[5] Notably, prescription pain relievers and heroin were also the main drugs associated with overdose deaths. In 2012, 259 million opioid prescriptions were written.[6] The rate of opioid overdoses tripled in the United States since 2000 to 28,647 deaths and accounted for 61% of all drug overdose deaths.[7] To counter the increasing number of opioid deaths, the Centers for Disease Control and Prevention (CDC) published practice guidelines in 2016 for safe prescribing of opioid medications for chronic pain conditions.[1]

Hypoventilation with terminal apnea is presumed to be a major of cause of death because many of these deaths reportedly occur during sleep, with no cause found at autopsy, except blood opioid levels. This article portrays the clinical features of opioid-induced sleep disordered breathing (SDB), investigates the potential pathophysiologic mechanisms for opioid-induced sleep apnea and provides the recent therapeutic advances for the treatment of chronic prescription opioid–induced SDB.

# CLINICAL MANIFESTATIONS
## Opioid-induced Sleep Disordered Breathing

SDB associated with opioids is distinct (**Fig. 1**) and has been extensively reviewed previously.[8–10] Briefly, these types of SDB include hypoventilation and, most commonly, mixed central and obstructive apneas and hypopneas. These events occur amid chaotic breathing patterns hitherto referred as ataxic breathing. This pattern is easily distinguished from the Hunter-Cheyne-Stokes breathing observed in patients with heart failure. In the background of ataxic breathing pattern, a cluster pattern and Biot breathing can be distinguished. Cluster breathing is characterized by cycles of deep breaths in which the amplitude of tidal volume is fairly stable with interspersed central apneas of variable durations. The Biot pattern is characterized by variable breathing rate and amplitude of tidal volume (discussed later).

## Central sleep apnea

It is well established that opioids cause ventilatory depression. Moreover, recent studies have established that patients receiving chronic opioid therapy for chronic pain have an increased

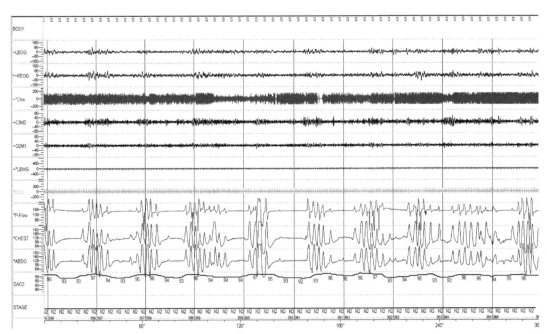

**Fig. 1.** A 5 minute-epoch of a polysomnogram showing obstructive (OSA) and central (CSA) apneas, and hypopneas in stage N2. There are repetitive central apneas with typical ataxic breathing pattern associated with opioids showing a mixture of Cluster and Biot's patterns. With CSA the airflow channels are flat associated with absence of effort on the thoraco-abdominal excursions. Also note fluctuations in SaO$_2$, which parallel the central apneas. Montage channels in descending order: body position, left electrooculogram (LEOG), right electrooculogram (REOG), chin electromyogram (EMG), central EEG, occipital EEG, leg EMG, pressure transducer, rib cage respiratory inductance plethysmography, abdomen respiratory inductance plethysmography, SaO$_2$, sleep stage.

prevalence of central sleep apnea (CSA).[11–17] Even a single dose of opioid analgesic acutely precipitated CSA in patients who had no underlying cardiac or neurologic disease or had preexisting obstructive sleep apnea (OSA).[16] Meanwhile, some studies showed a preponderance of obstructive apneas[18] or a combination of OSA and CSA (**Table 1**).

An early study comparing 50 stable methadone maintenance treatment (MMT) patients and 20 age-matched, sex-matched, and body mass index (BMI)–matched normal subjects noted that 30% (n = 15) of MMT patients had CSA, defined as a central apnea index (CAI) greater than 5/h.[11] These patients were compared with normal subjects (CAI<1/h). Central apneas and hypopneas occurred more often in the opioid users during non–rapid eye movement (NREM) sleep but not in rapid eye movement (REM) sleep,[11,19] a distribution pattern similar to that in heart failure.[20]

A retrospective study compared 60 patients on chronic opioids with mean morphine equivalent dose (MEQ) of 144 mg and median MEQ 79 mg, with 60 matched controls.[13] Compared with controls, the apnea-hypopnea index (AHI) was increased in the opioid group (44/h vs 30/h; P<.05) because of increased central apneas (13/h vs 2/h; P<.001). Within the opioid group, and after controlling for BMI, age, and sex, there was a dose-response relationship between MEQ and apnea-hypopnea (P<.001), obstructive apnea (P<.001), hypopnea (P<.001), and central apnea indices (P<.001). Ataxic or irregular breathing during NREM sleep was also more prevalent in patients who chronically used opioids (70% vs 5%; P<.001) and more frequent (92%) at an MEQ of 200 mg or higher (odds ratio = 15; P = .017).[13] Additional use of hypnotics did not seem to increase the risk for apneas and hypopneas in this population. In the only prospective study of 70 consecutive patients on buprenorphine, a semisynthetic μ-agonist used for opioid dependency, Farney and colleagues[17] observed primarily CSA (see **Table 1**).

As noted earlier, central apneas characteristically are dispersed in an ataxic[20] breathing pattern, including Biot breathing or cluster pattern with short cycle time.[13] Biot breathing is an ataxic breathing pattern with breaths of differing amplitude, without any regular rhythm, and with random apneic periods of variable duration[21] (see **Fig. 1**). This pattern is similar to the irregular breathing pattern observed after ablation of the pre-Bötzinger complex (preBötC) in the rat model[22] but is distinct from Hunter-Cheyne-Stokes breathing seen in patients with heart failure and characterized by waxing and waning breathing and long cycle time (>40 seconds). Most studies show the ataxic breathing at much lower doses of opioids.[11]

### Obstructive sleep apnea
Most studies show a preponderance of central apneas or a mix of central and obstructive events (see **Table 1**). However, in one study that did not include a control group, OSA (35%) rather than CSA (14%) was observed in a subset of MMT patients with poor sleep quality.[18] In another study,[23] 42 consecutive chronic mixed opioid users underwent full-night attended polysomnography. Investigators reported a high prevalence of OSA with an AHI of 44/h of sleep and CAI of 0.6/h. Thirty-one of the 42 patients had severe OSA with AHI greater than or equal to 30/h of sleep. Moreover, in a separate study, chronic opioid use was associated with positive airway pressure (PAP)–emergent CSA, a condition in which patients with OSA develop CSA on continuous positive airway pressure (CPAP) and the CSA persists in spite of long-term CPAP use.[24]

### Hypoventilation
*Hypoventilation while awake* While awake, severe diurnal hypoventilation is unusual in patients who use opioids chronically. In 50 patients on chronic methadone treatment, only 10 patients had a $Pa_{CO_2}$ between 45 and 50 mm Hg, with the remainder having normal arterial blood gas values.[25] In a separate study with chronic opioid use for pain control, 9 of 20 (45%) patients had daytime hypercapnia[26] (**Table 2**).

*Hypoventilation during sleep* Sleep and opioids share profound destabilizing effects on breathing and these adverse effects can become additive or synergistic.[27] Both opioids and sleep decrease hypercapnic ventilatory response (HCVR) and at the same time reduce upper airway muscle activity. The combination of increased upper airway resistance and reduced HCVR can lead to sustained hypoventilation and hypoxemia. Importantly, if diurnal hypercapnia is already present, in view of the combined effects of opioids and sleep reducing ventilation, the reduced ventilation should have a profound effect in increasing $P_{CO_2}$, as dictated by the alveolar ventilation equation, $Pa_{CO_2} = k \times V_{CO_2}/VA$, where $V_{CO_2}$ is $CO_2$ production and $VA$ is alveolar ventilation. In view of Dalton' s law, $P_{O_2}$ deceases considerably.[28]

Thus, significant oxygen desaturation was noted in several studies during sleep in chronic prescription opioid users compared with control groups.[11,13,16,29] MMT patients had a lower oxygen saturation ($Sp_{O_2}$) nadir than control subjects (91.5% ± 3.3% vs 93.1%± 2.5%; P<.059).[11]

**Table 1**
**Demographics and sleep disordered breathing parameters with chronic prescription opioid use**

| Study | Age (y) | Gender | BMI (kg/m²) | MEQ (mg) Range (Mean) | PSG Parameters (per hour or %) |
|---|---|---|---|---|---|
| Teichtahl et al,[29] 2001; prospective cross-sectional | 33 ± 6 | 6 M, 4 F | 27 ± 6 | 187.5–450 | AHI 20.4 ± 20.7 CAI 12.4 ± 15.5 OAI 0.7 ± 2.1 Nadir Sao₂ 90 ± 4 |
| Wang et al,[11] 2005; prospective cross-sectional | 35 ± 9 | 25 M, 25 F | 27 ± 6 | Not reported; methadone blood concentration: 0.34 ± 0.34 mg/L | AHI 17.5 ± 17.3 CAI 6.7 ± 14.2 OSAHI 10.8 ± 10.3 Nadir Sao₂ 91.5 ± 3.3 |
| Walker et al,[13] 2007; retrospective | 52.7 ± 13.1 | 20 M, 40 F | 31.8 ± 7.7 | 7.5–750 (143.9) | AHI 43.5 ± 35.2 CAI 12.8 ± 22.4 OAI 16.8 ± 24.0 Mean Sao₂ 89.3 ± 7.0 Ataxic breathing in 70% |
| Webster et al,[15] 2008; prospective cross-sectional | Mean 51 | N = 140, NA | 29.7 | 15–5985 (266) | AHI 75% CA 24% OA 39% No sleep apnea 25% |
| Mogri et al,[16] 2009; retrospective | 22–80 | M/F 1.39 | 20.7–47.3 | 7.5–935 (median 180) | SDB 85% CSA 24% OSA 36% Combined 31% Hypoxemia in 72% SDB No sleep apnea 15% |
| Sharkey et al,[18] 2010; prospective cross-sectional | 37.7 ± 8.1 | 29 M, 42 F | 28.4 ± 6.0 | 25–310 (108.3 ± 53.9) | CSA 14% OSA 35% |
| Jungquist et al,[76] 2012; prospective cross-sectional | 49.6 ± 12.4 | 25 M, 39 F | 33.9 ± 7.4 | 5–960 | AHI 22.7 ± 25 CAI 5.0 ± 13 OAI 4.4 ± 9 Nadir Sao₂ 83.5 ± 6 |
| Farney et al,[17] 2013; prospective cross-sectional | 31.8 ± 12.3 | 28 M, 42 F | 24.9 ± 5.9 | Buprenorphine dose 2.0–76.0 (18.5 ± 13.0) | AHI 20.4 ± 32 CAI 11.4 ± 28.1 OAI 2.3 ± 3.9 %TST Sao₂ <90% 23.2 ± 32.5; Biot breathing |
| Farney et al,[63] 2008; prospective cross-sectional | 50.1 ± 12.6 | 9 M, 13 F | 32.9 ± 6.1 | Not reported | AHI 66.6 ± 37.3 CAI 26.4 ± 25.1 OAI 25.8 ± 23. HI 14.5 ± 14.5 Nadir Spo₂ 79.5 ± 8.1 Biot breathing |
| Javaheri et al,[77] 2008; case series | 51 ± 4 | 4 M, 1 F | 31 ± 4 | 120–450 (252 ± 150) | AHI 70 ± 19 CAI 26 ± 27 OAI 6 ± 7 HI 1 ± 1 Nadir Sao₂ 86 ± 4 |

(continued on next page)

**Table 1**
*(continued)*

| Study | Age (y) | Gender | BMI (kg/m²) | MEQ (mg) Range (Mean) | PSG Parameters (per hour or %) |
|---|---|---|---|---|---|
| Alattar et al,[67] 2009; case series | 56.2 ± 10.7 | 2 M, 4 F | 33.2 ± 2.3 | 120–420, 272 ± 98 | AHI 51.5 ± 27.7 CA% total: 70 ± 16 Time with Sao$_2$ <90% 1.8 min to 6.4 h |
| Guilleminault et al,[23] 2010; retrospective | 45.9 ± 7.1 | 22 M, 22 F | 25.6 ± 1.9 | Doses not provided as MEQ | AHI 43.9 ± 5.2 CAI 0.6 ± 1.4 Mixed and obstructive HI 43.2 ± 3.1 |
| Chowdhuri et al,[66] 2012; retrospective | 53.7 ± 11.5 | 41 M | 33.9 ± 7.4 | 93 ± 102, median 40 | AHI 77.4 ± 33.1 CAI 37.6 ± 28.9 Nadir Sao$_2$ 80.5% ± 5.5%, |
| Ramar et al,[65] 2012; retrospective | 59.1 ± 14.2 | 23 M, 24 F | 33.9 ± 8.0 | Not reported | AHI 48.4 ± 33.3 CAI 17.8 ± 24.6 OAI 13.2 ± 19.9 |
| Rose et al,[26] 2010; prospective | 52.4 ± 9.4 | 12 M, 12 F | 34.9 ± 9.4 | 141 ± 97, median 120 | AHI 32.7 ± 25.6 CAI 3.9 ± 8.3 OAI 3.0 ± 6.0 HI 26.0 ± 20.5 %TST Sao$_2$ <90% 10.4 ± 17.6 |
| Javaheri et al,[31] 2014; prospective | 53 ± 10 | 13 M, 7 F | 33 ± 7 | 15–915, median 118 | AHI 61 ± 30 CAI 32 ± 31 OAI 5 ± 5 Nadir Sao$_2$ 83 ± 8 |
| Troitino et al,[19] 2014; retrospective | 60.8 ± 8.9 | N = 34 | 31.2 ± 3.6 | 30–217 (68) | AHI 45 ± 30.6 CAI 29.3 ± 22.6 OSAI 12.3 ± 9.4 Nadir Sao$_2$ 81.7 ± 8.1 %TST Sao$_2$ <90% 41.8 ± 25.1 |
| Shapiro et al,[78] 2015; prospective | 50.7 ± 11.6 | 11 M, 28 F | 30.1 ± 5.4 | 100–1700 (390.1 ± 338.1) | AHI 38.8 ± 31.1 CAI 16.1 ± 18.8 OSAI 9.7 ± 15.2 HI 14.8 ± 12.6 Nadir Sao$_2$ 79.9 ± 7.8 |

*Abbreviations:* AHI, apnea-hypopnea index; BMI, body mass index; CA, central apneas; CAI, central apnea index; F, female; HI, hypopnea index; M, male; MEQ, morphine equivalent dose; NA, not applicable; OSAI, obstructive sleep apnea index; PSG, polysomnography; Sao$_2$, oxygen saturation; %TST, percentage total sleep time.

Spo$_2$ in the opioid group was significantly lower than controls during both wakefulness (difference 2.1%; *P*<.001) and NREM sleep (difference 2.2%; *P*<.001).[13] Compared with healthy controls, chronic opioid users also had significantly higher percentage sleep time with Spo$_2$ less than 90% (10.4% ± 17.6% vs 0.1% ± 0.3%) and average desaturations (4.0% ± 1.4% vs 2.4% ± 0.8%).[26] This finding may indicate global hypoventilation and/or abnormal lung function with ventilation-perfusion mismatch. Of note, abnormal pulmonary function tests were observed among patients receiving long-term opioid therapy.[25] However, most MMT patients were also tobacco smokers.[25] In a sample of 50 MMT patients, diffusion capacity was reduced in 62%,[25] forced expiratory volume in 1 second was reduced in 17%, and 18% had an obstructive ventilatory defect, whereas the

**Table 2**
**Awake arterial blood gas parameters with chronic opioids**

| Study | Age (y) | Gender | BMI (kg/m²) | MEQ (mg) | ABG Results |
|-------|---------|--------|-------------|----------|-------------|
| Javaheri et al,[31] 2014 | 53 ± 10 | 13 M, 7 F | 33 ± 7 | Range 15–915, median 118, n = 7 | pH 7.36–7.42 $Paco_2$ 42–48 $Pao_2$ 80 (59–99) |
| Teichtachl et al,[25] 2004 | 35 ± 9 | 25 M, 25 F | 27 + 6 | Not reported | pH 7.40 ± 0.03 $Paco_2$ 42.2 ± 3.8 $Pao_2$ 81.4 ± 9.9 20% had $Paco_2$ of 45–50 mm Hg |
| Rose et al,[26] 2014 | 52.4 ± 9.4 | 12 M, 12 F | 34.9 ± 9.4 | Mean 141 ± 97, median 120 | pH 7.39 ± 0.02 $Paco_2$ 44.8 ± 4.1 $Pao_2$ 81.4 ± 9.9 |

Abbreviations: ABG, arterial blood gas; BMI, body mass index; MEQ, morphine equivalent dose.

alveolar-arterial $PaO_2$ difference was increased in 28%, in the absence of obvious underlying lung or cardiac disease.[25] In spite of adverse additive/synergistic effects of sleep and opioids on breathing, creating the perfect conditions for hypoventilation and potential for demise, no systematic studies are available to show the magnitude and the severity of hypoventilation in patients on chronic opioids with or without hypercapnia.[27]

### Effects on Sleep Architecture

Overall, accurate scoring of polysomnograms of patients on opioids is deemed difficult, because there may be large number of alpha waves intruding into the sleep architecture. MMT patients had significantly low sleep efficiency; decreased slow wave sleep,[29] REM sleep, and stage N1 sleep; and more N2 sleep compared with the normal subjects.[11,29] The MMT patients also tended to have longer sleep onset latency, higher arousal index, and less total sleep time than normal subjects.[25] In addition, the MMT patients had significantly more daytime sleepiness compared with the normal subjects as measured by the Epworth Sleepiness Scale.[19] One study described the effects on sleep of a single dose of oral opioid medication (sustained-release morphine sulfate 15 mg vs methadone 5 mg), given in a double-blind crossover fashion to 42 healthy patients without sleep apnea or chronic pain.[30] Both opioid drugs significantly reduced slow wave sleep and increased stage N2 sleep. However, neither drug had an effect on sleep efficiency, wake after sleep onset, or total sleep time. There was also no significant reduction in REM sleep.[30] In a study of 20 patients with SDB who underwent full-night attended polysomnography before and after therapy,[31] sleep efficiency was mildly reduced, with excessive stage N1, reduced stage REM, and a virtual absence of stage N3. Patients had severe sleep apnea with AHI 60/h and arousal index of 30/h of sleep. Overnight therapy with adaptive servoventilation attenuated the SDB resulting in improved sleep architecture with major reduction in stage N1 and arousals, and increased stage N2. Stage REM sleep did not change significantly.[31]

### PATHOPHYSIOLOGY OF OPIOID-INDUCED SLEEP DISORDERED BREATHING

Like beta agonists, opioid molecules act on the superfamily of G protein–coupled receptors. The opioid-specific receptor is a μ (mu) receptor that is prevalent at various neuronal sites involved in control of breathing. However, in contrast with beta agonists, opioids via μ receptors decrease intracellular cyclic AMP levels and depress respiratory neuronal function. Respiratory depression by opioids may manifest during wakefulness or while asleep (global hypoventilation with hypercapnia), and CSA and OSA.

### Effect on the pre-Bötzinger Complex and the Hypoglossal Motor Neuron Nucleus

The preBötC, the presumed site of respiratory rhythm genesis, is located in the ventral medullary respiratory column caudal to the Bötzinger nucleus.[32] Opioids are thought to bind to the μ receptors in the preBötC to depress the rate and depth of respiration,[33,34] which can be reversed by naloxone.[35,36] However, other studies failed to show the same effect of naloxone at the preBötC[37] and indicate that the reduced hypoxic ventilatory response of opioids occurs at the mu receptors of the nucleus tractus solitarius.[38]

The other major adverse effect of opioids on breathing during sleep has to do with reduction in genioglossus muscle activity, which can predispose to upper airway closure and obstructive SDB. There seem to be neuronal aggregates where opioids exert such an effect. In rodents these include the hypoglossal motor neuron pools[39]; the other is an aggregate of neurons close to the preBötC.[35] Animal studies show that opioids can significantly decrease hypoglossal nerve activity, leading to suppression of genioglossus muscle activity and potentially causing upper airway obstruction[39]; however, this has not yet been established in humans. Such effects are most pronounced during sleep and with the use of anesthetics.

In one of the earliest studies, the investigators measured the pressure generated by the first 0.1 second of inspiratory effort against a closed airway ($P_{0.1}$), in response to hypercapnia and hypoxia, with and without added inspiratory resistance, before and after oral meperidine.[40] With both hypercapnia and hypoxia, meperidine decreased the augmentation of $P_{0.1}$ that was associated with increased resistance. Thus, normal individuals respond to acute increases of inspiratory resistance by increasing inspiratory motor output but this increase was blunted by meperidine.[40] As noted earlier, administration of the μ-opioid receptor agonist, fentanyl, at the hypoglossal motor neuron caused the suppression of genioglossus muscle activity that was reversed by the μ-opioid receptor antagonist, naloxone.[39] In humans, naloxone reduced upper airway collapsibility in normal sleeping patients following sleep fragmentation.[41] This finding may explain abnormal upper airway function in adult and pediatric patients with OSA perioperatively and postoperatively in the presence of μ-opioid analgesics.[42]

### Effect on Chemoresponsiveness

Human studies have shown that acute administration of opioid drugs causes dose-dependent bradypnea, reduced tidal volume, impaired pulmonary gas exchange, and blunting of ventilatory responsiveness to hypoxia and hypercapnia during wakefulness.[43] The hypoxic ventilatory response (HVR) decreased 60% from $108 \pm 17$ to $43 \pm 5$ L/min/mm Hg, whereas the hypercapnic ventilatory response (HCVR) decreased 42% from $1.69 \pm 0.24$ to $0.98 \pm 0.20$ L/min/mm Hg, 45 to 60 minutes following a single subcutaneous dose of 7.5 mg of morphine sulfate in 6 healthy adult men, indicating decreased ventilatory responsiveness.[43] This study provides the important clinical implication that narcotics contribute to acute ventilatory depression and

hypoventilation. However, in healthy individuals without sleep apnea who were given a single dose of oral hydromorphone, there was no significant change in the HCVR or pharyngeal resistance.[44] The HVR decreased significantly from $0.65 \pm 0.17$ to $0.56 \pm 0.15$ ($P<.05$) but without an associated change in the number of apneas or hypopneas during sleep following hydromorphone.[44]

Although opioids decrease ventilatory responsiveness acutely[43,44] this does not seem to be the case following chronic use,[45] suggesting there may be development of tolerance to methadone. In this single study, in patients in an MMT program on chronic oral methadone, there was a significant decline in the HCVR ($1.27 \pm 0.61$ L/min/mm Hg vs $1.64 \pm 0.57$ L/min/mm Hg; $P<.05$) compared with controls, but an increase rather than a decrease in the HVR ($2.14 \pm 1.58$ L/min/% arterial oxygen saturation vs $1.12 \pm 0.7$; $P<.05$), the latter potentially suggestive of the presence of increased peripheral chemoresponsiveness.[45] The ventilatory changes were related to changes in respiratory rate rather than tidal volume. The mechanism of this disparate finding with chronic versus acute opioid use remains unclear but it can be speculated that hypoxia during sleep from chronic opioid use may potentiate peripheral chemoresponsiveness with increase in the controller gain (ie, increase in the slope of ventilatory responsiveness). In addition, MMT patients with an antidepressant in the blood had significantly reduced HCVR compared with patients without ($0.83 \pm 0.59$ L/min/mm Hg vs $1.34 \pm 0.59$ L/min/mm Hg; $P<.05$). Thus, it is conceivable that, during sleep, narcotics blunt central chemoresponsiveness, contributing to increased steady-state $P_{CO_2}$ (ie, increased plant gain [a measure of the eupneic drive to breathe]).[46,47] However, if there is also increased HVR with chronic opioid use,[45] the controller gain could be increased.[46] Thus a combination of increased controller and plant gains (both are components of loop gain) may potentially increase the slope of $CO_2$ chemosensitivity below eupnea, reducing the carbon-dioxide reserve (carbon-dioxide reserve = difference between eupneic $CO_2$ and apneic threshold $CO_2$), in which narrowing of the $CO_2$ reserve precipitates breathing instability, resulting in repetitive apneas and hypopneas during sleep[47] (**Fig. 2**).

Chronic opioid use blunts hypercapnic responsiveness,[48] predisposing to hypoventilation, particularly during sleep and after anesthesia, when upper airway resistance is increased. Newborns, the elderly, postoperative patients and those with chronic obstructive pulmonary disease, those with SDB, or those who are high risk for SDB

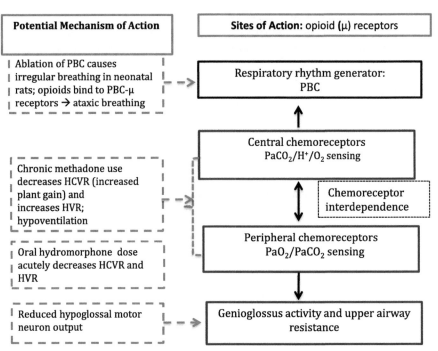

**Fig. 2.** The potential pathways of opioid-induced SDB. The μ opioid receptors at different sites provide targets for potential therapies.

should be most susceptible to the effects of opioids.[49–52] Of note, there are no studies directly investigating chemoreceptor control of breathing during sleep in patients with either acute or chronic opioid intake.

Animal studies suggest that opioids tonically depress the respiratory network. The opioid receptor blocker, naloxone, stimulated respiratory output in anesthetized, normoxic, normocapnic cats[53] and in unanesthetized hypoxic or hypercapnic animals.[54] In contrast, in awake human adults, naloxone does not affect ventilation. In a randomized, double-blind, placebo-controlled study of 13 normal subjects, intravenous injection of naloxone (0.1 mg/kg) had no significant effect on baseline ventilation or ventilatory response to isocapnic hypoxia.[55] Similarly, in another randomized placebo-controlled study in 12 healthy men, intravenous administration of naloxone (10 mg) did not affect the slopes or x-intercepts of the relationships between either minute ventilation or $P_{0.1}$ and arterial $O_2$ during progressive isocapnic HVR.[56] In contrast, endorphins have an inhibitory effect in the central respiratory response to hypercapnia but hypoxic ventilatory depression does not seem to be mediated by endorphins in adults.[57] However, a randomized study suggested modulation of the hypercapnic ventilatory response by endogenous opioids that was reversed by naloxone.[55]

## CLINICAL OUTCOMES

As noted earlier, there has been increasing mortality with increasing use of prescription chronic opioids. A large number of young individuals on opioids are found dead in bed and at autopsy no cause is found, except opioids and other drugs such as benzodiazepines in the blood (death-in-bed syndrome). A report indicated that SDB might play a role in unexplained excess mortality in patients treated with methadone.[58] However, there are no records on the exact mechanisms of death. Hypoventilation and SDB resulting in fatal hypoxia, hypercapnic acidosis, and a terminal apnea should be sine qua non of death. Studies also noted that patients with chronic opioid use were sleepier, had poor reaction times, and had poorer sleep quality[18,26] than patients without chronic opioid use.

## THERAPEUTIC STRATEGIES FOR OPIOID-INDUCED SLEEP DISORDERED BREATHING

There are multiple approaches for treatment of SDB associated with the use of opioids.[59,60] Prevention is the most important step for this public health problem. However, in most cases the presence of ongoing chronic pain precludes this option. Thus, no standardized therapies exist for SDB associated with opioid use. Empiric PAP-based therapies have been attempted (see **Table 1**). These therapies include CPAP with and without supplemental oxygen, bilevel PAP (BPAP) with and without backup respiratory rate, and adaptive servoventilation (ASV), with varying effects on resolution of SDB. However, the impact of these PAP-based therapies on morbidity and mortality in patients with opioid-induced SDB is not known. More recently, animal and human studies show that therapy based on a neurotransmitter, ampakine, may effectively treat opioid-induced sleep apnea.

## Opioid Detoxification

The CDC has provided recommendations for minimizing opioid dosing to prevent toxicity and overdose. The guideline suggests that clinicians should "avoid prescribing opioids to patients with moderate or severe SDB whenever possible to minimize risks for opioid overdose."[1] The most appropriate intervention for treatment of sleep apnea was related to opioid use. Three studies have shown that detoxification reverses central and perhaps obstructive SDB.[9,61,62]

## Treatment of Opioid-related Central Sleep Apnea

### Positive airway pressure therapy

Four retrospective and 2 prospective studies have evaluated the effect of PAP/ASV therapy on SDB occurring in patients with opioid use (**Table 3**). The studies had small sample sizes, variable definitions of CSA and titration success, and variable demographics. Three studies did not report opioid dosing or did not convert doses to morphine equivalent dosing. Farney and colleagues[63] reported a high percentage of ataxic Biot respiration in patients with SDB related to chronic opioid use and noted a remarkable lack of success with either CPAP or ASV therapy (see **Table 3**). The current ASV devices use different algorithms to restore minute ventilation, or peak airflow when there is a reduction to less than 90% to 95% of the baseline,[64] which is accomplished by adjusting inspiratory pressure support. The automatic backup rate algorithm aborts any impending apnea by delivering a mandatory breath.

Ramar and colleagues[65] and Troitino and colleagues[19] reported successful ASV titration in 60%, whereas Javaheri and colleagues[31] reported success with ASV in 100% of their patients. Appropriate pressure selection of these devices is critical to success.[8] CPAP also showed variable success rates, from 0%[31] to 24%[19] to 54%.[66] Chowdhuri and colleagues[66] also described the use of adjunctive supplemental oxygen therapy with PAP in patients with residual CSA on CPAP. However, in 1 study,[48] addition of supplemental oxygen did not correct SDB and associated hypoxia.

One study used a multimodality strategy with addition of supplemental oxygen during CPAP or BPAP titration after CPAP alone did not eliminate repetitive central apneas.[66] BPAP with backup rate also reduced SDB in a small case series.[67] Javaheri and colleagues[31] noted absence of response to CPAP despite 2 attempts at CPAP titration at intervals of 4 to 8 weeks. In contrast, ASV was effective with CSA at baseline as well as with PAP-emergent CSA in patients with chronic opioid–induced SDB.[31] The mean ASV adherence for these patients was 5.1 ± 2.5 hours per night at follow-up. However, adherence was poor in a study by Troitino and colleagues,[19] in which only 18% of patients were adherent to ASV at 12 months.

Cao and colleagues[68] randomized patients to BPAP with a backup rate (bilevel-ST [spontaneous-timed]) versus ASV with autotitrating expiratory PAP (auto-EPAP) and found that ASV achieved significantly higher levels of correction of sleep apnea compared with BPAP with a backup rate of 9.1 ± 2.9. Respiratory parameters were normalized in 83.3% of participants on ASV versus 33.3% on bilevel-ST but there were no significant differences in the average oxygen saturation (%) or minimum oxygen saturation (%). Total sleep time was significantly higher with bilevel-ST compared with ASVauto without any difference in the sleep efficiency or sleep architecture.[68]

### Acetazolamide

Acetazolamide is a respiratory stimulant and is effective in the treatment of CSA. In a randomized double-blind trial, overnight administration of acetazolamide significantly decreased CAI in patients with heart failure.[69] This effect is likely mediated by reductions in the plant gain and the sensitivity below eupnea.[46] A case report of a young woman on long-acting opioids and OSA described the development of CSA on CPAP that was unresponsive to supplemental oxygen.[70] After addition of an oral nightly dose of 250 mg of acetazolamide, optimal CPAP was obtained during a repeat titration study. However, there are no systematic studies of the effects of acetazolamide or other pharmacologic agents that may work by altering chemoreceptor control of breathing of opioid-induced SDB.

### Ampakines

Several pharmacologic agents have been used experimentally to stabilize respiration in animals.[71] One such agent, AMPA (amino-3-hydroxy-5-methyl-D-aspartate) receptor agonist (ampakine),

**Table 3**
**Impact of positive airway pressure therapy with opioid-related sleep disordered breathing**

| Study | MEQ (mg) | Study Design and Population | Therapeutic Success on PAP (Defined as AHI <10/h and CAI <5/h in Some Studies*) | | |
|---|---|---|---|---|---|
| | | | CPAP | BPAP | ASV |
| Alattar & Scharf,[67] 2009 | 120–420 | Retrospective, CSA, n = 5 | 1 out of 5 One patient responded to CPAP of 20 cm $H_2O$ | 3 out of 4 with BPAP-ST, backup rate but hypoxia persisted | NA |
| Farney et al,[63] 2008 | Not reported | Retrospective; n = 22 | 6% (1 out of 18); moderate or severe Biot respiration noted in 94% of patients on CPAP | NA | 0 (0 out of 22); moderate to severe Biot respiration in 82% of patients on ASV |
| Guilleminault et al,[23] 2010 | MEQ not provided, individual opioid doses provided | Retrospective, n = 44 | AHI on CPAP: 13.81 ± 2.77/h | AHI on BPAP: 11.52 ± 2.12/h BPAP with backup rate: 1.70 ± 0.58/h | NA |
| Ramar et al,[65] 2012* | Not reported | Retrospective; CSA and PAP-emergent CSA, n = 47 | NA | NA | 60% (28 out of 47) ASV |
| Chowdhuri et al,[66] 2012* | 93 ± 102, median 40 | Retrospective, veterans, excluded PAP-emergent CSA, n = 41 | CPAP 54% (22 out of 41) CPAP and adjunctive $O_2$ 27% (11 out of 41) | BPAP and adjunctive $O_2$ 10% (4 out of 41), no backup rate | NA |
| Troitino et al,[19] 2014* | 68 (30–217) | Retrospective, veterans, n = 34 | 24% (8 out of 34) | 66% (6 out of 9), backup rate 15/min | 60% (12 out of 20) ASV |
| Javaheri et al,[31] 2014 | 15–915, median = 118 | Prospective, nonrandomized; CSA and PAP-emergent CSA, n = 18 | 0 out of 16 (0%) | NA | CAI <5/h: 100% (20 out of 20) with ASV |
| Cao et al,[68] 2014 | MEQ not provided, individual opioid doses provided | Randomized crossover; CSA, unclear if PAP-emergent CSA was included, n = 18 in each arm | 4 out of 5 | 33% normalized with BPAP-ST + backup rate | ASV with auto-EPAP, 83% normalized with ASV |
| Shapiro et al,[78] 2015 | 100–1700 (390.1 ± 338.1) | Prospective, randomized crossover | CPAP AHI 10.1 (17.4 ± 20.1), n = 31 | ASV AHI 1.4 (4.5 ± 7.3), n = 31 | ASV with PSmin 6, AHI 2.1 (7.6 ± 16.7), n = 31 |

*Abbreviations:* BPAP-ST, spontaneous (S mode) timed mode (T mode); auto-EPAP, autotitrating expiratory PAP; PSmin, pressure support, minimum.

when administered to the pre-Bötzinger area, countered the respiratory depressant effects of opioid drugs without affecting their analgesic effects.[34,72] Specifically, the ampakine CX717 administered to rats countered fentanyl-induced respiratory depression without significantly altering analgesia and sedation, or the animals' behavior.[73] Both ventilatory depression and analgesia were reversed with naloxone. Human studies have shown reversal of opioid-induced respiratory depression by ampakines.[74,75] In 16 healthy men, after a single oral dose of 1500 mg of the ampakine CX717 and an opioid drug, alfentanil, respiratory frequency was decreased by $2.9\% \pm 33.4\%$ compared with a decrease in respiratory rate by $25.6\% \pm 27.9\%$ when coadministered with placebo ($P<.01$).[75] Blood oxygenation and the ventilatory response to hypercapnic challenge also showed significantly smaller decreases with CX717 than with placebo. In contrast, CX717 did not affect alfentanil-induced analgesia. Randomized clinical trials are needed to determine whether ampakines play any role in the treatment of opioid-induced CSA.

### Treatment of Opioid-related Obstructive Sleep Apnea

#### Positive airway pressure therapy

The treatment of choice for OSA associated with opioids presumably is CPAP; however, in 1 study of 50 patients with OSA treated with CPAP, central apneas emerged,[23] and were eliminated with the use of a bilevel device with a backup rate. Of note, most studies alluded to earlier had a combination of CSA and OSA with variable responses to PAP (see **Table 3**).

### RESEARCH AGENDA

Evidence is limited as to the effects of chronic opioid use on control of breathing during wakefulness and sleep and several questions related to the prevalence and impact of chronic opioid use remain unanswered. Optimal treatment strategies also need to be investigated in depth. Thus, to address these gaps in knowledge, the authors suggest the following research goals:

1. Establish the prevalence of OSA and CSA in patients with chronic opioid use.
2. Determine the dose and frequency at which different opioid drugs induce SDB.
3. Determine what is the least detrimental dose of opioids in patients with and without underlying SDB.
4. Determine whether the presence of SDB in patients with chronic opioid is associated with

adverse clinical outcomes, including death, cardiovascular events, and neurocognitive dysfunction.
5. Determine whether antidepressants and benzodiazepines alter the effects of acute and chronic opioid use on the above outcomes.
6. Delineate the exact pathophysiology of opioid-induced sleep apnea in humans. Does chronic opioid use increase HVR while concomitantly decreasing HCVR during sleep?
7. Initiate pathophysiology-guided therapies for opioid-induced SDB.
8. Investigate the role of ampakines alone or in combination with PAP and oxygen therapy for the treatment of opioid-related SDB in patients with underlying OSA.
9. Determine the long-term effects on sleep, cardiovascular outcomes, and neurocognitive outcomes of novel ampakine-based therapies in patients with chronic opioid use.

### SUMMARY

Opioid-induced SDB presents a therapeutic predicament with the increasing incidence of prescription opioid use for noncancer chronic pain in the United States. CSA with a Biot or cluster breathing pattern is characteristic of polysomnography studies; however, long-term clinical outcomes and the impact of therapy remain unknown. Novel ampakine-based therapies are being investigated. Randomized controlled trials with therapies that target the underlying pathophysiologic mechanisms of opioid-induced SDB are required.

### REFERENCES

1. Centers for Disease Control and Prevention. CDC guideline for prescribing opioids for chronic pain—United States, 2016. MMWR Recomm Rep 2016; 65(1):1–49.
2. Nahin RL. Estimates of pain prevalence and severity in adults: United States, 2012. J Pain 2015;16(8):769–80.
3. Institute of Medicine. Relieving pain in America: a blueprint for transforming prevention, care, education, and research. Washington, DC: The National Academies Press; 2011.
4. Chou R, Fanciullo GJ, Fine PG, et al. Clinical guidelines for the use of chronic opioid therapy in chronic noncancer pain. J Pain 2009;10(2):113–30.e2.
5. Boudreau D, Von Korff M, Rutter CM, et al. Trends in de-facto long-term opioid therapy for chronic noncancer pain. Pharmacoepidemiol Drug Saf 2009; 18(12):1166–75.
6. Centers for Disease Control and Prevention. Opioid painkiller prescribing, where you live makes a

difference. 2014. Available at: http://www.cdc.gov/vitalsigns/opioid-prescribing/. Accessed November 14, 2016.

7. Rudd RA, Aleshire N, Zibbell JE, et al. Increases in drug and opioid overdose deaths–United States, 2000-2014. MMWR Morb Mortal Wkly Rep 2016; 64(50):1378–82.

8. Javaheri S, Brown L, Randerath W. Positive airway pressure therapy with adaptive servo ventilation (part II: clinical applications). Chest 2014;10:637–43.

9. Javaheri S, Patel S. Opioids cause central sleep apnea in humans. Am J Respir Crit Care Med 2016; 193:A4222.

10. Cao M, Javaheri S. Chronic opioid use: effects on respiration and sleep. Edited by Nova Science Publishers, Inc. Opioids pharmacology, clinical uses and adverse effects. New York: 2012. 1–13.

11. Wang D, Teichtahl H, Drummer O, et al. Central sleep apnea in stable methadone maintenance treatment patients. Chest 2005;128(3):1348–56.

12. Wang D, Teichtahl H. Opioids, sleep architecture and sleep-disordered breathing. Sleep Med Rev 2007;11(1):35–46.

13. Walker JM, Farney RJ, Rhondeau SM, et al. Chronic opioid use is a risk factor for the development of central sleep apnea and ataxic breathing. J Clin Sleep Med 2007;3(5):455–61.

14. Correa D, Farney RJ, Chung F, et al. Chronic opioid use and central sleep apnea: a review of the prevalence, mechanisms, and perioperative considerations. Anesth Analg 2015;120(6):1273–85.

15. Webster LR, Choi Y, Desai H, et al. Sleep-disordered breathing and chronic opioid therapy. Pain Med 2008;9(4):425–32.

16. Mogri M, Desai H, Webster L, et al. Hypoxemia in patients on chronic opiate therapy with and without sleep apnea. Sleep Breath 2009;13(1):49–57.

17. Farney RJ, McDonald AM, Boyle KM, et al. Sleep disordered breathing in patients receiving therapy with buprenorphine/naloxone. Eur Respir J 2013; 42(2):394–403.

18. Sharkey KM, Kurth ME, Anderson BJ, et al. Obstructive sleep apnea is more common than central sleep apnea in methadone maintenance patients with subjective sleep complaints. Drug Alcohol Depend 2010;108(1):77–83.

19. Troitino A, Labedi N, Kufel T, et al. Positive airway pressure therapy in patients with opioid-related central sleep apnea. Sleep Breath 2014;18(2):367–73.

20. Javaheri S, Parker T, Liming J, et al. Sleep apnea in 81 ambulatory male patients with stable heart failure types and their prevalences, consequences, and presentations. Circulation 1998;97(21):2154–9.

21. Biot M. Contribution a l'etude du phenomene respiratoire de Cheyne-Stokes. Lyon Med 1876;23:517–28, 561–7.

22. McKay LC, Janczewski WA, Feldman JL. Sleep-disordered breathing after targeted ablation of pre-Bötzinger complex neurons. Nat Neurosci 2005; 8(9):1142.

23. Guilleminault C, Cao M, Yue HJ, et al. Obstructive sleep apnea and chronic opioid use. Lung 2010; 188(6):459–68.

24. Javaheri S, Smith J, Chung E. The prevalence and natural history of complex sleep apnea. J Clin Sleep Med 2009;5(3):205.

25. Teichtahl H, Wang D, Cunnington D, et al. Cardiorespiratory function in stable methadone maintenance treatment (MMT) patients. Addict Biol 2004;9(3–4): 247–53.

26. Rose AR, Catcheside PG, McEvoy RD, et al. Sleep disordered breathing and chronic respiratory failure in patients with chronic pain on long term opioid therapy. J Clin Sleep Med 2014;10(8):847–52.

27. Arora N, Cao M, Javaheri S. Opioids, sedatives, and sleep hypoventilation. Sleep Med Clin 2014;9(3): 391–8.

28. Javaheri S. Determinants of carbon dioxide tension. In: Gennari FJ, Adrogue HJ, Gall JH, et al, editors. Acid-base disorders and their treatment. Boca Raton (FL): Taylor and Francis; 2005. p. 47–77.

29. Teichtahl H, Prodromidis A, Miller B, et al. Sleep-disordered breathing in stable methadone programme patients: a pilot study. Addiction 2001; 96(3):395–403.

30. Dimsdale JE, Norman D, DeJardin D, et al. The effect of opioids on sleep architecture. J Clin Sleep Med 2007;3(1):33–6.

31. Javaheri S, Harris N, Howard J, et al. Adaptive servoventilation for treatment of opioid-associated central sleep apnea. J Clin Sleep Med 2014; 10(6):637–43.

32. Smith JC, Ellenberger HH, Ballanyi K, et al. Pre-Botzinger complex: a brainstem region that may generate respiratory rhythm in mammals. Science 1991;254(5032):726–9.

33. Janczewski WA, Onimaru H, Homma I, et al. Opioid-resistant respiratory pathway from the preinspiratory neurones to abdominal muscles: in vivo and in vitro study in the newborn rat. J Physiol 2002;545(3): 1017–26.

34. Greer JJ, Carter JE, Al-Zubaidy Z. Opioid depression of respiration in neonatal rats. J Physiol 1995; 485(3):845–55.

35. Montandon G, Qin W, Liu H, et al. PreBötzinger complex neurokinin-1 receptor-expressing neurons mediate opioid-induced respiratory depression. J Neurosci 2011;31(4):1292–301.

36. Montandon G, Horner R. CrossTalk proposal: the preBotzinger complex is essential for the respiratory depression following systemic administration of opioid analgesics. J Physiol 2014;592(6): 1159–62.

37. Mustapic S, Radocaj T, Sanchez A, et al. Clinically relevant infusion rates of mu-opioid agonist remifentanil cause bradypnea in decerebrate dogs but not via direct effects in the pre-Botzinger complex region. J Neurophysiol 2010;103(1):409–18.

38. Zhang Z, Zhang C, Zhou M, et al. Activation of opioid mu-receptors, but not delta- or kappa-receptors, switches pulmonary C-fiber-mediated rapid shallow breathing into an apnea in anesthetized rats. Respir Physiol Neurobiol 2012;183(3):211–7.

39. Hajiha M, DuBord MA, Liu H, et al. Opioid receptor mechanisms at the hypoglossal motor pool and effects on tongue muscle activity in vivo. J Physiol 2009;587(Pt 11):2677–92.

40. Kryger MH, Yacoub O, Dosman J, et al. Effect of meperidine on occlusion pressure responses to hypercapnia and hypoxia with and without external inspiratory resistance. Am Rev Respir Dis 1976; 114(2):333–40.

41. Meurice J-C, Marc I, Series F. Effects of naloxone on upper airway collapsibility in normal sleeping subjects. Thorax 1996;51(8):851–2.

42. Lam KK, Kunder S, Wong J, et al. Obstructive sleep apnea, pain, and opioids: is the riddle solved? Curr Opin Anaesthesiol 2016;29(1):134–40.

43. Weil JV, McCullough RE, Kline J, et al. Diminished ventilatory response to hypoxia and hypercapnia after morphine in normal man. N Engl J Med 1975; 292(21):1103–6.

44. Robinson RW, Zwillich CW, Bixler EO, et al. Effects of oral narcotics on sleep-disordered breathing in healthy adults. Chest 1987;91(2):197–203.

45. Teichtahl H, Wang D, Cunnington D, et al. Ventilatory responses to hypoxia and hypercapnia in stable methadone maintenance treatment patients. Chest 2005;128(3):1339–47.

46. Nakayama H, Smith CA, Rodman JR, et al. Effect of ventilatory drive on carbon dioxide sensitivity below eupnea during sleep. Am J Respir Crit Care Med 2002;165(9):1251–60.

47. Dempsey JA. Crossing the apnoeic threshold: causes and consequences. Exp Physiol 2005; 90(1):13–24.

48. Santiago TV, Edelman N. Opioids and breathing. J Appl Physiol (1985) 1985;59(6):1675–85.

49. Moss I, Scott S, Inman J. Hypoxia, sleep and respiration in relation to opioids in developing swine. Respir Physiol 1993;92(1):115–25.

50. Taylor S, Kirton OC, Staff I, et al. Postoperative day one: a high risk period for respiratory events. Am J Surg 2005;190(5):752–6.

51. Moss IR, Laferrière A. Central neuropeptide systems and respiratory control during development. Respir Physiol Neurobiol 2002;131(1):15–27.

52. Zhang C, Moss IR. Age-related mu-, delta- and kappa-opioid ligands in respiratory-related brain regions of piglets: effect of prenatal cocaine. Brain Res Dev Brain Res 1995;87(2):188–93.

53. Lawson EE, Waldrop TG, Eldridge FL. Naloxone enhances respiratory output in cats. J Appl Physiol Respir Environ Exerc Physiol 1979;47(5): 1105–11.

54. Schlenker EH, Inamdar SR. Effects of naloxone on oxygen consumption and ventilation in awake golden Syrian hamsters. Physiol Behav 1995;57(4): 655–8.

55. Tabona M, Ambrosino N, Barnes PJ. Endogenous opiates and the control of breathing in normal subjects and patients with chronic airflow obstruction. Thorax 1982;37(11):834–9.

56. Steinbrook RA, Weinberger SE, Carr DB, et al. Endogenous opioids and ventilatory responses to hypoxia in normal humans 1–4. Am Rev Respir Dis 1985;131(4):588–91.

57. Kagawa S, Stafford MJ, Waggener TB, et al. No effect of naloxone on hypoxia-induced ventilatory depression in adults. J Appl Physiol Respir Environ Exerc Physiol 1982;52(4):1030–4.

58. Porucznik CA, Farney RJ, Walker JM, et al. Increased mortality rate associated with prescribed opioid medications: is there a link with sleep disordered breathing? Eur Respir J 2005;26:596 (abstract).

59. Javaheri S, Randerath WJ. Opioid-induced central sleep apnea: mechanisms and therapies. Sleep Med Clin 2014;9(1):49–56.

60. Javaheri S, Germany R, Greer JJ. Novel therapies for the treatment of central sleep apnea. Sleep Med Clin 2016;11(2):227–39.

61. Ramar K. Reversal of sleep-disordered breathing with opioid withdrawal. Pain Pract 2009;9(5): 394–8.

62. Davis MJ, Livingston M, Scharf SM. Reversal of central sleep apnea following discontinuation of opioids. J Clin Sleep Med 2012;8(5):579.

63. Farney RJ, Walker JM, Boyle KM, et al. Adaptive servoventilation (ASV) in patients with sleep disordered breathing associated with chronic opioid medications for non-malignant pain. J Clin Sleep Med 2008;4(4):311–9.

64. Javaheri S, Brown LK, Randerath WJ. Positive airway pressure therapy with adaptive servoventilation: part 1: operational algorithms. Chest 2014; 146(2):514–23.

65. Ramar K, Ramar P, Morgenthaler TI. Adaptive servoventilation in patients with central or complex sleep apnea related to chronic opioid use and congestive heart failure. J Clin Sleep Med 2012; 8(5):569.

66. Chowdhuri S, Ghabsha A, Sinha P, et al. Treatment of central sleep apnea in US veterans. J Clin Sleep Med 2012;8(5):555–63.

67. Alattar MA, Scharf SM. Opioid-associated central sleep apnea: a case series. Sleep Breath 2009; 13(2):201–6.

68. Cao M, Cardell C, Willes L, et al. A novel adaptive servoventilation (ASVAuto) for the treatment of central sleep apnea associated with chronic use of opioids. J Clin Sleep Med 2014;10(8): 855–61.

69. Javaheri S. Acetazolamide improves central sleep apnea in heart failure: a double-blind, prospective study. Am J Respir Crit Care Med 2006;173(2): 234–7.

70. Glidewell RN, Orr WC, Imes N. Acetazolamide as an adjunct to CPAP treatment: a case of complex sleep apnea in a patient on long-acting opioid therapy. J Clin Sleep Med 2009;5(1):63–4.

71. Dempsey JA, Veasey SC, Morgan BJ, et al. Pathophysiology of sleep apnea. Physiol Rev 2010;90: 47–112 [Erratum appears in Physiol Rev 2010; 90(2):797–8].

72. Ren J, Poon BY, Tang Y, et al. Ampakines alleviate respiratory depression in rats. Am J Respir Crit Care Med 2006;174(12):1384–91.

73. Greer JJ, Ren J. Ampakine therapy to counter fentanyl-induced respiratory depression. Respir Physiol Neurobiol 2009;168(1–2):153–7.

74. Van Der Schier R, Roozekrans M, Van Velzen M, et al. Opioid-induced respiratory depression: reversal by non-opioid drugs. F1000Prime Rep 2013;6:79.

75. Oertel B, Felden L, Tran P, et al. Selective antagonism of opioid-induced ventilatory depression by an ampakine molecule in humans without loss of opioid analgesia. Clin Pharmacol Ther 2010;87(2): 204–11.

76. Jungquist CR, Flannery M, Perlis ML, et al. Relationship of chronic pain and opioid use with respiratory disturbance during sleep. Pain Manag Nurs 2012; 13(2):70–9.

77. Javaheri S, Malik A, Smith J, et al. Adaptive pressure support servoventilation: a novel treatment for sleep apnea associated with use of opioids. J Clin Sleep Med 2008;4(4):305–10.

78. Shapiro CM, Chung SA, Wylie PE, et al. Home-use servo-ventilation therapy in chronic pain patients with central sleep apnea: initial and 3-month follow-up. Sleep Breath 2015;19(4):1285–92.

# Obesity Hypoventilation Syndrome
## Choosing the Appropriate Treatment of a Heterogeneous Disorder

Amanda J. Piper, PhD[a,b,*], Ahmed S. BaHammam, MD[c,d], Shahrokh Javaheri, MD[e,f,g]

**KEYWORDS**

- Obesity hypoventilation syndrome • Continuous positive airway pressure • Hypercapnia
- Nocturnal hypoventilation • Sleep disordered breathing

**KEY POINTS**

- Obesity hypoventilation syndrome (OHS) covers a spectrum of sleep breathing abnormalities from predominantly repetitive obstructive apneas, combined obstructive apneas with sleep hypoventilation, or isolated sleep hypoventilation.
- There is no strong evidence to recommend one form of positive airway pressure (PAP) therapy over another in terms of clinical outcomes in OHS with concomitant obstructive sleep apnea.
- Response to PAP seems to be influenced by adherence to therapy and the OHS phenotype being treated.
- Cardiovascular risk remains high despite effective PAP therapy.
- Weight loss and reduced sedentary behavior are important components of a comprehensive management program for these individuals.

## BACKGROUND

Obesity hypoventilation syndrome (OHS) is characterized by chronic awake hypercapnia ($Paco_2$ >45 mm Hg, at sea level) and sleep disordered breathing in obese individuals (body mass index [BMI] >30 kg/m$^{-2}$) in the absence of any other explanations for chronic hypercapnia.[1–3] When Burwell and colleagues[4] first described this condition as a Pickwickian syndrome, treatment options were limited: weight loss, tracheostomy, and short-term respiratory stimulants. The key contribution of sleep disordered breathing to

Disclosure statement: A.J. Piper has received lecture fees from ResMed Australia and Philips Respironics, manufacturers of positive airway pressure (PAP) devices. She also received grant money from the ResMed Foundation to conduct a trial evaluating PAP therapy in obesity hypoventilation syndrome. A.S. BaHammam and S. Javaheri report no conflict of interest.

[a] Sleep Unit, Department of Respiratory and Sleep Medicine, Royal Prince Alfred Hospital, Missenden Road, Camperdown, New South Wales 2050, Australia; [b] Central Medical School, University of Sydney, Sydney 2006, New South Wales, Australia; [c] The University Sleep Disorders Center, Department of Medicine, College of Medicine, King Saud University, Riyadh 11324, Saudi Arabia; [d] National Plan for Science and Technology, King Saud University, Riyadh 11324, Saudi Arabia; [e] Montgomery Sleep Laboratory, Bethesda North Hospital, Cincinnati, OH 45242, USA; [f] Pulmonary and Sleep Medicine, University of Cincinnati, Cincinnati, OH, USA; [g] Division of Cardiology, Ohio State University, Columbus, OH, USA

* Corresponding author. Sleep Unit, Department of Respiratory and Sleep Medicine, Royal Prince Alfred Hospital, Missenden Road, Camperdown, New South Wales 2050, Australia.
E-mail address: amanda.piper@sydney.edu.au

Sleep Med Clin 12 (2017) 587–596
http://dx.doi.org/10.1016/j.jsmc.2017.07.008
1556-407X/17/© 2017 Elsevier Inc. All rights reserved.

the evolution of this syndrome was not appreciated. Although one of the earliest reports of continuous positive airway pressure (CPAP) for sleep disordered breathing involved 2 patients with OHS achieving reversal of their awake respiratory failure with nocturnal therapy,[5] over the next 2 decades few studies addressed the management of these individuals in a systematic manner. However, in the last 10 years increasing global obesity rates[6] in conjunction with a growing appreciation of the high health care costs,[7] morbidity and mortality associated with OHS,[8–10] has increased interest in the early diagnosis and effective treatment of this disorder.[1,11]

The development of awake hypercapnia in OHS is the culmination of a complex interplay of factors, the mix of which varies from individual to individual: reduced lung volumes, decreased respiratory system compliance, increased upper airway resistance during wakefulness and sleep, lack of augmented drive to compensate for obesity, impaired inspiratory muscle performance, and reduced chemoreceptor sensitivity to hypercapnia and hypoxia.[12] However, sleep disordered breathing is universally present, ranging from repetitive obstructive apneas to prolonged obstructive or nonobstructive hypopneic breathing, most marked during periods of rapid eye movement sleep.[13] Moderate to severe obstructive sleep apnea (OSA) occurs in most patients with OHS, with the sleep hypoventilation phenotype occurring in 10% to 15% of individuals.[14,15]

Normalizing nocturnal breathing and gas exchange is the goal of positive airway pressure (PAP) therapy. In OHS this involves maintaining upper airway patency, improving alveolar ventilation, reducing the work of breathing, and eliminating hypoxemia. Given the heterogeneity of sleep breathing abnormalities seen within and between individuals with OHS, different PAP therapies may be variously successful depending on the clinical phenotype and clinical setting (**Table 1**).

## MODES OF POSITIVE AIRWAY PRESSURE THERAPY

By providing a single level of pressure throughout the respiratory cycle, CPAP does not directly improve hypercapnia through augmentation of ventilation. Nevertheless, it addresses several other mechanisms contributing to abnormal breathing during sleep. By stabilizing the upper airway and eliminating repetitive obstructive events, CPAP attenuates the cycle of low ventilation during apneic periods and consequent

hypoxemic burden, carbon dioxide ($CO_2$) accumulation, and longer-term bicarbonate retention.[16] In addition, by increasing lung volumes, airway resistance and flow limitation are reduced, contributing to a reduction in the work of breathing, especially when recumbent.[17] Improvements in oxygenation could also be expected through the prevention of acute hypercapnia and small airway closure and improved ventilation-perfusion inequality. However, CPAP will not overcome the work of breathing arising from obesity-induced reductions in chest wall compliance.[18]

Bilevel PAP (BPAP) therapy provides 2 levels of pressure, with the expiratory (EPAP) component providing the same effects as CPAP therapy in addition to active augmentation of tidal volume ($V_T$) through its inspiratory component (IPAP). Both the spontaneous and spontaneous-timed (ST) modes of BPAP have been used in OHS, with the latter being recommended in the presence of central apneas, whereby respiratory rates are inappropriately low or whereby minute ventilation remains reduced.[19] In patients with stable OHS, the spontaneous mode (BPAP-S) has been associated with a significant increase in respiratory events, mainly of central and mixed origin, compared with the ST mode.[20] This increase is likely due to the augmented ventilation, lowering the prevailing $P_{CO_2}$ to less than the apneic threshold $P_{CO_2}$ resulting in cessation of breathing. Conversely, patient-ventilator asynchrony and discomfort have been described with BPAP-ST.[20,21] However, using the ST mode with a higher backup rate to achieve more passive ventilation (less patient triggering) may produce more stable breathing[20] with greater improvements in awake $CO_2$ levels.[22]

A limitation of fixed level pressure support (BPAP) is the variability of delivered $V_T$ due to changes in respiratory effort, respiratory system compliance and sleep position in patients with OHS. Volume-targeted pressure support (VtPS) combines the advantages of pressure-limited and volume-limited modes of ventilation into one mode in order to achieve adequate $V_T$ and minute ventilation throughout a sleep period and long-term.[23] A built-in pneumotachograph monitors delivered $V_T$ and when $V_T$ drops to less than a preset threshold, the device automatically responds by increasing IPAP (pressure support) to augment $V_T$ to approach the target $V_T$ (**Fig. 1**). In many of the newer devices, EPAP can be set to automatically adjust in response to obstructive events. Most randomized studies comparing PAP modes in OHS have included VtPS as one of the therapy arms.[15,22,24–27]

**Table 1**
**Overview of positive airway pressure therapies for obesity hypoventilation syndrome**

| PAP Mode | Uses and Benefits | Comments |
|---|---|---|
| CPAP | • Suitable as initial therapy trial in patients with stable OHS with moderate to severe OSA<br>• Can be considered in some patients after initial stabilization with BPAP<br>• Least costly of all PAP therapy | • Pressures 10–16 cm $H_2O$ generally required<br>• Improvement in awake gas exchange over the first month may be slower compared with BPAP modes<br>• Lack of long-term comparative data with other modes of PAP |
| BPAP-spontaneous | • Suitable for patients with good drive and ability to trigger consistently to IPAP in all sleep stages<br>• Less expensive than spontaneous-timed modes of PAP | • Limited comparative data with other PAP modes<br>• May induce central events if not titrated correctly |
| BPAP–spontaneous-timed | • Widely used in acute and home settings<br>• First-line therapy for patients with isolated nocturnal hypoventilation<br>• Can be set to provide a minimum rate or to achieve passive ventilation | • Patient-ventilator asynchrony can persist and impact on efficacy<br>• Also recommended when respiratory rate remains low or minute ventilation is reduced despite best pressure support |
| BPAP with volume-targeted pressure support | • Should provide more stable ventilation by targeting a predetermined tidal volume<br>• Adapts to changes in sleep stage, posture, and lung mechanics on a continuous basis | • Variable air leaks and persisting airway obstruction may reduce efficacy<br>• Should reduce the need for manual titration of pressures<br>• No evidence of additional clinical benefits compared with other PAP modes |

*Abbreviations:* BPAP, bilevel PAP; IPAP, inspiratory PAP.

## POSITIVE AIRWAY PRESSURE THERAPY AND STABLE ACUTE HYPERCAPNIC RESPIRATORY FAILURE

Clinically, 50% to 80% of ambulatory patients with stable OHS with concomitant OSA will respond to CPAP therapy either during the first titration night or over a period of weeks to months of continued CPAP use.[8,28–30] Reliably distinguishing a priori CPAP responders from nonresponders is not possible; though not surprisingly, those with more severe upper airway obstruction, less sleep time spent with $SpO_2$ less than 90%, less severe obesity, and better preserved vital capacity are more likely to be effectively managed with CPAP alone.[30–32] In contrast to long-term observational data of BPAP-treated OHS,[33,34] few studies have reported on CPAP-treated OHS beyond 3 months.[8,35]

Both CPAP and BPAP therapy have been shown to be more effective than lifestyle modification in improving nocturnal oxygenation, sleep quality, and awake hypercapnia in patients with OHS with OSA over a 1- to 2-month period.[26,36] A 3-month study comparing patients with stable OHS randomly allocated to CPAP or BPAP-S mode found no between-group differences in change in awake $Pa_{CO_2}$, hours of therapy usage, health-related quality of life (HRQoL), or daytime sleepiness.[29] However, small differences in perceived sleep quality and psychomotor vigilance favoring BPAP were reported. Interpretation of the study findings are limited by the exclusion of patients who continued to have sustained desaturation ($SpO_2$ <80% for >10 minutes) on best titrated CPAP levels for safety reasons and the use of the spontaneous mode, which may have

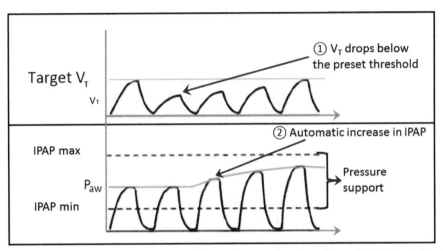

**Fig. 1.** The principles of operation of VtPS mode. When $V_T$ drops to less than the set $V_T$ ①, the device detects the drop in $V_T$ and automatically increases IPAP (pressure support) to restore $V_T$ to the target $V_T$ ②.

provided less efficient ventilation compared with ST modes of support.[20]

In a subsequent multicenter randomized study comparing CPAP with fixed level BPAP-ST over 3 months, no difference in the proportion of participants with treatment failure (defined by hospital admission, persistent or worsening ventilatory failure, or nonadherence) was seen over a 3-month period.[18] Similar improvements in Paco₂ and bicarbonate after 1 and 3 months of treatment occurred in each group, although there was a trend toward a more rapid decrease in Paco₂ at the first month with BPAP-ST. No between-group differences in other secondary outcomes, including sleepiness, HRQoL, cardiovascular risk markers, physical activity, or sedentary behavior, occurred. In the largest randomized controlled trial so far reported, Masa and colleagues[26] randomized 221 patients with OHS associated with severe OSA into 3 arms: lifestyle modification (1000-calorie diet, regular sleep habits, exercise, and avoiding sedatives, stimulants, alcohol, and smoking tobacco), CPAP, or BPAP-ST with VtPS (both combined with lifestyle modification). The main outcome was the change in Paco₂. At 2 months, all treatment arms showed improvement in hypercarbia. Decrements in Paco₂ were 5.5, 3.7, and 3.2 mm Hg, with BPAP in VtPS mode, CPAP, and lifestyle modifications, respectively. Reduction in Paco₂ was greatest with assured ventilation and significantly different from the control arm but not the CPAP arm. For this reason, the investigators thought that CPAP should be considered the first-line treatment of OHS associated with OSA, to which the authors also agree. Improvements in vital capacity and 6-minute walk distance favored the BPAP group, although the clinical relevance of

the small differences in these secondary outcomes are unclear given the short period of observation.

Most studies have compared BPAP-ST mode with BPAP-ST with VtPS.[22,24–27] In these studies, the addition of VtPS led to higher IPAP levels with higher $V_T$[25,27] or minute ventilation[24] producing significantly greater reductions in overnight CO₂.[25,27] However, the improved nocturnal ventilation with VtPS did not seem to provide any additional HRQoL benefits.[27] Murphy and colleagues[22] randomized 50 patients with stable OHS to BPAP-ST with or without VtPS over a 3-month period and similarly found no additional benefit from VtPS in terms of improved daytime gas exchange, symptoms, HRQoL, or activity levels. Unlike the earlier studies, these investigators titrated both BPAP modes to achieve a prespecified CO₂ target, demonstrating similar levels of delivered pressure support produce similar clinical outcomes. Current evidence does not support any significant benefits of VtPS over fixed pressure BPAP or CPAP, although it may be useful in selected cases.

A synthesis of the available data regarding PAP therapies for stable OHS with OSA suggests that the response to therapy is influenced not so much by PAP mode but rather the extent to which nocturnal ventilation and gas exchange are controlled (**Table 2**). Consequently, for cost and simplicity, CPAP may be used for most patients with OHS with OSA as initial therapy or following a period of stabilization on BPAP (**Fig. 2**). Importantly, adherence to therapy is a significant modifier of PAP response[28]; every effort should be made to encourage more than 4.0 to 4.5 hours' nightly use.[22,28]

**Table 2**
Randomized trials of short-term home positive airway pressure therapy in patients with obesity hypoventilation syndrome and obstructive sleep apnea

| Author | Masa et al,[26] 2015 (Spain) | | | Borel et al,[36] 2012 (France) | | Piper et al,[29] 2008 (Australia) | | Howard et al,[18] 2017 (Australia) | | Murphy et al,[22] 2012 (England) | |
|---|---|---|---|---|---|---|---|---|---|---|---|
| Therapy | Lifestyle | CPAP | Bilevel ST (V$_T$PS) | Lifestyle | Bilevel ST | CPAP | Bilevel S | CPAP | Bilevel ST | Bilevel ST | Bilevel ST (V$_T$PS) |
| Study period (mo) | | 2 | | | 1 | | 3 | | 3 | | 3 |
| Subjects (n) | 70 | 80 | 71 | 18 | 19 | 18 | 18 | 31 | 29 | 25 | 25 |
| M:F | 31:39 | 42:38 | 25:46 | 7:11 | 8:11 | 14:4 | 9:9 | 18:13 | 14:15 | 11:14 | 12:13 |
| Age (y) | 60 (13) | 57 (13) | 64 (11) | 54 (6) | 58 (11) | 52 (17) | 47 (13) | 52 (10) | 53 (11) | 56 (11) | 53 (9) |
| BMI, kg/m$^{-2}$ | 44 (7) | 45 (8) | 43 (7) | 40 (4) | 40 (6) | 52 (7) | 54 (9) | 54 (11) | 55 (13) | 52 (8) | 50 (8) |
| Baseline Paco$_2$ (mm Hg) | 51.0 (4.2) | 50.0 (4.5) | 51.0 (4.3) | 45 (3) | 48.0 (4.5) | 52 (49–55) | 49 (47–57) | 52 (6) | 50 (5) | 51 (6) | 52 (5) |
| Baseline FVC (% predicted) | 82 (20) | 80 (20) | 78 (19) | 88 (14) | 79 (21) | 62 (14) | 64 (20) | 57 (17) | 62 (18) | 56 (15) | 52 (14) |
| IPAP (cm H$_2$O) | NA | NA | 20 | NA | 18 (3) | NA | 16 (2) | NA | 19 (3) | 23 (4) | 22 (5) |
| CPAP/EPAP (cm H$_2$O) | NA | 11 | 7.8 | NA | 11 (2) | 14 (3) | 10 (2) | 15 (3) | 12 (2) | 10 (2) | 9 (1) |
| ΔPaco$_2$ (mm Hg) | −3.2 (6.0) | −3.7 (6.6) | −5.5 (7.0) | −1.4 | −4.9 | −5.8 (8.4) | −6.9 (6.7) | 6.2 | 5.8 | −4.5 (8.25) | −4.5 (7.5) |
| Wt loss kg | −1.6 (5.0) | −1.1 (5.6) | −2.4 (6.6) | — | — | −4.9 (7.8) | −5.6 (9.4) | — | — | — | — |
| ΔBMI | — | — | — | −0.4 | 0 | — | — | −2.1 | −1.1 | −2 (4) | −1 (2) |
| Compliance (h per night) | NA | 5.3 (2.1) | 5.3 (2.3) | NA | 5.6 (2.2) | 5.8 (2.4) | 6.1 (2.1) | 5.0 (2.4) | 5.3 (2.6) | 5.08 (2.2) | 4.11 (2.5) |

*Abbreviations:* F, female; FVC, forced vital capacity; M, male; NA, not applicable; Wt, weight.

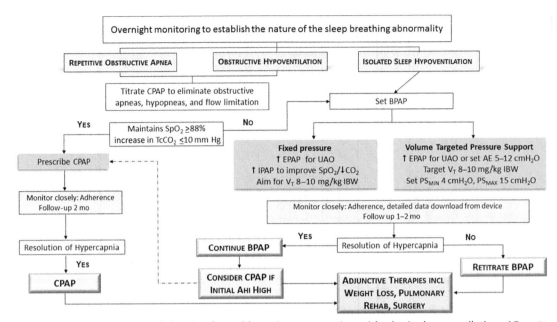

**Fig. 2.** PAP therapy choice and titration for stable patients presenting with obesity hypoventilation. AE, auto-EPAP; AHI, apnea hypopnea index; IBW, ideal body weight; INCL, including; $PS_{MAX}$, maximum pressure support; $PS_{MIN}$, minimum pressure support; $TcCO_2$, transcutaneous carbon dioxide; UAO, upper airway obstruction.

The impact of PAP therapy in patients with OHS without OSA has received less attention. An observational study looking at longer-term outcomes compared OHS phenotypes with and without OSA. All were treated with BPAP-ST. Improvements in awake blood gases and lung function were similar between groups, although there was a trend toward better survival in those with concomitant OSA. More recently, a multicenter trial from Spain randomized 86 patients to 2 months of lifestyle modification alone (a 1000-calorie diet and sleep advice) or in conjunction with BPAP-ST with VtPS.[15] Over this short time period, more significant improvements in awake $Paco_2$ and bicarbonate levels, daytime sleepiness, and nocturnal breathing were seen in the BPAP group.

## POSITIVE AIRWAY PRESSURE THERAPY IN ACUTELY DECOMPENSATED OBESITY HYPOVENTILATION SYNDROME

Obesity hypoventilation syndrome remains under-recognized as a cause of acute hypercapnic respiratory failure (AHRF). Up to 40% of patients with OHS present for the first time with AHRF,[22,37–39] yet less than one-third may receive the correct diagnosis during their admission.[10,40] Early recognition and treatment are vital, as patients with OHS admitted with AHRF have a high rate of in-hospital mortality (18%).[40] PAP therapy, commonly with the addition of controlled supplemental oxygen,

is the mainstay therapy for hospitalized patients with OHS and AHRF.[41]

Although PAP therapy is frequently used in acute decompensated OHS, there are no randomized trials comparing the efficacy of different modes of therapy. Current guidelines recommend starting BPAP therapy in these patients using the same blood gas criteria and precautions as in patients with acute exacerbations of chronic obstructive pulmonary disease[42] (**Box 1**). Therapy should also be commenced before performing a sleep study, because early initiation of PAP therapy may obviate invasive mechanical ventilation.[43] However, once stable and acid-base imbalance is corrected, patients may be shifted to CPAP with titration under polysomnographic monitoring.[43] **Table 3** outlines the proposed schema for initiating BPAP for patients with OHS with AHRF. Noninvasive ventilation (NIV) plays an important role in the management of these patients because intubation is at times quite difficult given the narrow airway of particularly morbidly obese patients. For the same reason, these patients may have severe obstructive events, particularly during sleep, necessitating requirement for high positive-end expiratory pressure. In addition, in order to augment ventilation, high inspiratory pressure support is required.

A prospective study of 76 patients examined factors associated with NIV failure in patients with OHS presenting with acute respiratory failure. Severe pneumonia and multiple organ failure often caused early NIV failure in those with hypoxemic respiratory failure.[44] In contrast, BPAP was more consistently successful for acute hypercapnic respiratory failure. Of note, more than half the patients experienced a delayed response to NIV, with persistence of hypercapnic acidosis during the first 6 hours.[44] These individuals were more likely to have received diuretics or respiratory depressant drugs before admission. Close and careful monitoring is needed to distinguish between the individual with a more prolonged response to BPAP but in whom therapy will be ultimately successful and the one who is failing therapy and requires intubation.

Patients with OHS presenting with acute respiratory failure generally have a more restrictive pulmonary defect and higher $Paco_2$ than those who commenced therapy during clinical stability.[22,39] Higher levels of EPAP[40] and pressure support[22] may be required in the acute setting compared with those used during clinical stability and may be a reason for patients failing to respond to therapy.[45]

## OXYGEN THERAPY

In patients with untreated stable OHS, moderate concentrations of oxygen administered during wakefulness worsens hypercapnia and acidemia as a consequence of hypoventilation and worsening dead space ventilation.[46] Oxygen breathing suppresses carotid bodies and hypoxic drive with consequent hypoventilation, while also reversing hypoxic-induced low ventilation/perfusion areas with consequent worsening dead space ventilation. For these reasons, nocturnal oxygen does not reduce $CO_2$ retention or daytime symptoms.[47]

As noted earlier, supplemental oxygen in addition to PAP is often needed during the early stages of treatment to maintain $SpO_2$ greater than 88%,

**Table 3**
A proposed schema for the management of acute hypercapnic respiratory failure in patients with obesity hypoventilation syndrome

| Indication for NIV in Acutely Decompensated OHS[42] | Commence BPAP Setup | Monitoring |
|---|---|---|
| pH <7.35, $Paco_2$ >45 mm Hg, RR >23 <br> Or <br> Daytime $Paco_2$ >49 mm Hg and somnolent <br> No contraindications to PAP therapy [Box 1] <br> Avoid administration of excessive levels of supplemental oxygen <br> Target $SpO_2$ 88%–92%[42] | - Appropriate mask fit to minimize leak/optimize comfort <br> - Set EPAP 4–6 cm $H_2O$, increasing in 1- to 2-cm $H_2O$ increments to eliminate <br>   - Witnessed apneas <br>   - Chest wall paradox <br>   - Snoring <br> - Set IPAP >6 cm $H_2O$ greater than EPAP to achieve adequate ventilation, targeting 8–10 mL/kg ideal body weight[22] <br> Careful titration of supplemental $O_2$[46] Consider positioning for upper airway obstruction | Close observation of <br> - $SpO_2$ <br> - Vital signs <br> - Level of consciousness <br> - Respiratory pattern <br> - $V_T$ <br> - Blood gases <br> Identify & treat reversible causes of AHRF, avoid excessive diuresis with loop diuretics[51] <br> Review use of medications with sedating or respiratory depressant effects[51] <br> - Consider IMV if BPAP fails <br> - Once stable, consider PSG and possible switch to CPAP and other long-term therapy[43] |

*Abbreviations:* IMV, invasive mechanical ventilation; NIV, noninvasive ventilation; PSG, polysomnogram.

although this can be withdrawn in many patients once effective and regular use of PAP therapy is achieved.[8,28,29,38] Baseline hypoxemia and the need of ongoing oxygen therapy in OHS are predictors of long-term mortality,[33,39] suggesting close follow-up in such patients is needed.

## IMPACT OF POSITIVE AIRWAY PRESSURE THERAPY ON CARDIOVASCULAR AND MORTALITY OUTCOMES

Controlled trials of PAP therapy in OHS have predominantly used change in awake $Paco_2$ as the primary measure of PAP efficacy. Other clinical and patient-centered outcomes, such as sleep quality, symptoms, and HRQoL, improve to a similar degree irrespective of the form of PAP used,[18,22,26,29] although these studies are likely to have been insufficiently powered to identify significant differences in secondary outcomes. There is evidence of improved functional capacity[15,26] and physical activity[18,22] following the use of PAP therapy as well as weight loss,[15,18,22,29] but it does not seem these changes produce clinically important benefits with respect to cardiovascular risk markers at least in the short-term.[18,36] Observational cohort studies suggest improved survival with PAP therapy, compared with historical controls,[33,48] although an increased risk of death compared with eucapnic OSA remains,[8] mainly associated with cardiovascular disease.[8,48]

## TITRATION OF POSITIVE AIRWAY PRESSURE THERAPY DURING SLEEP

During CPAP titration, pressure is progressively increased to a level that eliminates apneas, hypopneas, and flow limitation,[49] with slightly higher exploratory pressures to ensure oxygenation has been maximized.[31]

There is no consensus regarding how BPAP is best titrated. In general, EPAP is set at an initial pressure of 4 to 6 cm $H_2O$ with IPAP at least 4 cm $H_2O$ higher. In some centers, EPAP and IPAP are then increased in parallel for apneic obstruction, with further increases in IPAP for hypopnea, flow limitation, snoring, and nonapneic hypoventilation.[26] In others, EPAP and IPAP are increased together for obstructive events (apneas, hypopneas, or snoring), with further increases in IPAP to prevent hypoventilation (assessed by $V_T$, transcutaneous $CO_2$, or sustained nonapneic desaturation).[18,22,29] This variation in the approach to managing respiratory events does not seem to impact greatly on daytime or sleep outcomes (see **Table 2**). Pressure support (IPAP – EPAP) should not be less than 4 cm $H_2O$, with a target of 8 to 10 mL/kg ideal body weight to effectively augment ventilation.[22] High inspiratory pressures are needed to provide adequate $V_T$ given the poor compliance of the respiratory system, particularly in morbidly obese individuals. Studies evaluating automated EPAP algorithms in comparison with manually titrated EPAP have not yet been published, but it will be of importance to see how these algorithms respond to the changing dynamics of obstructive events with time and whether this impacts clinical outcomes.

## SEX DIFFERENCES IN OBESITY HYPOVENTILATION SYNDROME AND RESPONSE TO POSITIVE AIRWAY PRESSURE

Recent data have indicated some sex differences in patients with OHS. Women with OHS are older, more obese, have more deranged blood gases, and have more comorbidities than men.[37,50] Moreover, among patients referred to sleep clinics with suspected OSA, OHS seems to be most prevalent in postmenopausal women than premenopausal women and men.[50] Women are also more likely to present with the clinical phenotype of OHS without associated OSA.[15,34] Presentation with acute decompensation is more common in women, suggesting OHS may be underrecognized in women.[37] In a Swedish national registry assessing sex differences in patients with OHS starting long-term home ventilation, the 5-year survival rate was 68% (95% confidence interval [CI], 63.6%–72.3%) in men versus 59% (95% CI, 54.2%–64.0%) in women.[37] However, after adjusting for age, no sex-related survival difference was observed. Likewise, a French study reported women with OHS had a lower risk of death; but again after adjusting for confounders, the sex difference was lost.[48] Finally, more women seem to present with OHS without OSA; but whether there is a difference in survival between the clinical phenotypes of OHS with and without OSA is unknown.[34]

## SUMMARY

The initial goal of the treatment of OHS is to effectively attenuate hypercapnia, improve hypoxemia, and control sleep disordered breathing. Most individuals with OHS will present in a stable state through sleep laboratories with concomitant OSA. In this group, CPAP either as initial therapy or after a short period of BPAP provides similar benefits to BPAP. In patients presenting with acute decompensated OHS BPAP with supplemental controlled oxygen is the therapy of choice. In those with OSA, a switch to CPAP is often possible once clinical stability has been achieved. Longer-term comparative studies looking at the impact of PAP on morbidity, health resource use, and mortality are currently underway[15,18,26] and will provide important information to guide clinical decisions around longer-term PAP management in OHS. Regardless of the results of these studies, it is clear that PAP therapy addresses only 2 aspects of OHS, namely, sleep disordered breathing and awake hypercapnia. Interventions that encourage long-term weight loss, increase physical activity, and reduce daily sedentary behavior are also needed to manage those aspects of the disorder arising from obesity and its complications.

## REFERENCES

1. Egea-Santaolalla C, Javaheri S. Obesity hypoventilation syndrome. Curr Sleep Med Rep 2016;2:12–9.
2. Javaheri S, Simbartl LA. Respiratory determinants of diurnal hypercapnia in obesity hypoventilation syndrome. What does weight have to do with it? Ann Am Thorac Soc 2014;11(6):945–50.
3. Mokhlesi B. Obesity hypoventilation syndrome: a state-of-the-art review. Respir Care 2010;55(10): 1347–62.
4. Burwell CS, Robin ED, Whaley RD, et al. Extreme obesity associated with alveolar hypoventilation; a Pickwickian syndrome. Am J Med 1956;21(5):811–8.
5. Sullivan CE, Berthon-Jones M, Issa FG. Remission of severe obesity-hypoventilation syndrome after short-term treatment during sleep with nasal continuous positive airway pressure. Am Rev Respir Dis 1983; 128(1):177–81.
6. NCD Risk Factor Collaboration (NCD-RisC). Trends in adult body-mass index in 200 countries from 1975 to 2014: a pooled analysis of 1698 population-based measurement studies with 19.2 million participants. Lancet 2016;387(10026):1377–96.
7. Jennum P, Kjellberg J. Health, social and economical consequences of sleep-disordered breathing: a controlled national study. Thorax 2011;66(7):560–6.
8. Castro-Añón O, Pérez de Llano LA, De la Fuente Sánchez S, et al. Obesity-hypoventilation syndrome: increased risk of death over sleep apnea syndrome. PLoS One 2015;10(2):e0117808.
9. Jennum P, Ibsen R, Kjellberg J. Morbidity prior to a diagnosis of sleep-disordered breathing: a controlled national study. J Clin Sleep Med 2013; 9(2):103–8.
10. Nowbar S, Burkart KM, Gonzales R, et al. Obesity-associated hypoventilation in hospitalized patients: prevalence, effects, and outcome. Am J Med 2004;116(1):1–7.
11. Piper A. Obesity hypoventilation syndrome: weighing in on therapy options. Chest 2016;149(3):856–68.
12. Piper AJ, Grunstein RR. Big breathing: the complex interaction of obesity, hypoventilation, weight loss, and respiratory function. J Appl Physiol (1985) 2010;108(1):199–205.
13. Berger KI, Ayappa I, Chatr-Amontri B, et al. Obesity hypoventilation syndrome as a spectrum of respiratory disturbances during sleep. Chest 2001;120(4): 1231–8.
14. Kessler R, Chaouat A, Schinkewitch P, et al. The obesity-hypoventilation syndrome revisited: a prospective study of 34 consecutive cases. Chest 2001;120(2):369–76.
15. Masa JF, Corral J, Caballero C, et al. Non-invasive ventilation in obesity hypoventilation syndrome without severe obstructive sleep apnoea. Thorax 2016;71(10):899–906.
16. Berger KI, Goldring RM, Rapoport DM. Obesity hypoventilation syndrome. Semin Respir Crit Care Med 2009;30:253–61.
17. Steier J, Jolley CJ, Seymour J, et al. Neural respiratory drive in obesity. Thorax 2009;64(8):719–25.
18. Howard M, Piper A, Stevens B, et al. A randomised controlled trial of CPAP versus non-invasive ventilation for initial treatment of obesity hypoventilation syndrome. Thorax 2017;72(5):437–44.
19. Berry R, Chediak A, Brown L, et al. Best clinical practices for the sleep center adjustment of noninvasive positive pressure ventilation (NPPV) in stable chronic alveolar hypoventilation syndromes. J Clin Sleep Med 2010;6(5):491–509.
20. Contal O, Adler D, Borel JC, et al. Impact of different back-up respiratory rates on the efficacy of non-invasive positive pressure ventilation in obesity hypoventilation syndrome: a randomized trial. Chest 2013;143(1):37–46.
21. Guo YF, Sforza E, Janssens JP. Respiratory patterns during sleep in obesity-hypoventilation patients treated with nocturnal pressure support: a preliminary report. Chest 2007;131(4):1090–9.
22. Murphy PB, Davidson C, Hind MD, et al. Volume targeted versus pressure support non-invasive ventilation in patients with super obesity and chronic respiratory failure: a randomised controlled trial. Thorax 2012;67(8):727–34.
23. Pluym M, Kabir AW, Gohar A. The use of volume-assured pressure support noninvasive ventilation in acute and chronic respiratory failure: a practical guide and literature review. Hosp Pract 2015;43(5): 299–307.
24. Ambrogio C, Lowman X, Kuo M, et al. Sleep and non-invasive ventilation in patients with chronic respiratory failure. Intensive Care Med 2009;35(2): 306–13.
25. Janssens JP, Metzger M, Sforza E. Impact of volume targeting on efficacy of bi-level non-invasive ventilation and sleep in obesity-hypoventilation. Respir Med 2009;103(2):165–72.

26. Masa JF, Corral J, Alonso ML, et al. Efficacy of different treatment alternatives for obesity hypoventilation syndrome: Pickwick study. Am J Respir Crit Care Med 2015;192(1):86–95.

27. Storre JH, Seuthe B, Fiechter R, et al. Average volume-assured pressure support in obesity hypoventilation: a randomized crossover trial. Chest 2006;130(3):815–21.

28. Mokhlesi B, Tulaimat A, Evans AT, et al. Impact of adherence with positive airway pressure therapy on hypercapnia in obstructive sleep apnea. J Clin Sleep Med 2006;2(1):57–62.

29. Piper AJ, Wang D, Yee BJ, et al. Randomised trial of CPAP vs bilevel support in the treatment of obesity hypoventilation syndrome without severe nocturnal desaturation. Thorax 2008;63(5):395–401.

30. Salord N, Mayos M, Miralda RM, et al. Continuous positive airway pressure in clinically stable patients with mild-to-moderate obesity hypoventilation syndrome and obstructive sleep apnoea. Respirology 2013;18(7):1135–42.

31. Banerjee D, Yee BJ, Piper AJ, et al. Obesity hypoventilation syndrome: hypoxemia during continuous positive airway pressure. Chest 2007;131(6):1678–84.

32. Perez de Llano LA, Golpe R, Ortiz Piquer M, et al. Clinical heterogeneity among patients with obesity hypoventilation syndrome: therapeutic implications. Respiration 2008;75(1):34–9.

33. Budweiser S, Riedl SG, Jorres RA, et al. Mortality and prognostic factors in patients with obesity-hypoventilation syndrome undergoing noninvasive ventilation. J Intern Med 2007;261(4):375–83.

34. Ojeda Castillejo E, de Lucas Ramos P, Lopez Martin S, et al. Noninvasive mechanical ventilation in patients with obesity hypoventilation syndrome. Long-term outcome and prognostic factors. Arch Bronconeumol 2015;51(2):61–8.

35. Hida W, Okabe S, Tatsumi K, et al. Nasal continuous positive airway pressure improves quality of life in obesity hypoventilation syndrome. Sleep Breath 2003;7(1):3–12.

36. Borel JC, Tamisier R, Gonzalez-Bermejo J, et al. Noninvasive ventilation in mild obesity hypoventilation syndrome: a randomized controlled trial. Chest 2012;141(3):692–702.

37. Palm A, Midgren B, Janson C, et al. Gender differences in patients starting long-term home mechanical ventilation due to obesity hypoventilation syndrome. Respir Med 2016;110:73–8.

38. Perez de Llano LA, Golpe R, Ortiz Piquer M, et al. Short-term and long-term effects of nasal intermittent positive pressure ventilation in patients with obesity-hypoventilation syndrome. Chest 2005;128(2):587–94.

39. Priou P, Hamel J-F, Person C, et al. Long-term outcome of noninvasive positive pressure ventilation for obesity hypoventilation syndrome. Chest 2010;138(1):84–90.

40. Marik PE, Desai H. Characteristics of patients with the "malignant obesity hypoventilation syndrome" admitted to an ICU. J Intensive Care Med 2013;28(2):124–30.

41. Carrillo A, Ferrer M, Gonzalez-Diaz G, et al. Noninvasive ventilation in acute hypercapnic respiratory failure caused by obesity hypoventilation syndrome and chronic obstructive pulmonary disease. Am J Respir Crit Care Med 2012;186(12):1279–85.

42. Davidson AC, Banham S, Elliott M, et al. BTS/ICS guideline for the ventilatory management of acute hypercapnic respiratory failure in adults. Thorax 2016;71(Suppl 2):ii1–35.

43. Bahammam AS, Al-Jawder SE. Managing acute respiratory decompensation in the morbidly obese. Respirology 2012;17(5):759–71.

44. Lemyze M, Taufour P, Duhamel A, et al. Determinants of noninvasive ventilation success or failure in morbidly obese patients in acute respiratory failure. PLoS One 2014;9(5):e97563.

45. Piper AJ. Obesity hypoventilation syndrome: the pressure for effective treatment. Minerva Pneumol 2014;53(3):105–17.

46. Hollier CA, Harmer AR, Maxwell LJ, et al. Moderate concentrations of supplemental oxygen worsen hypercapnia in obesity hypoventilation syndrome: a randomised crossover study. Thorax 2014;69(4):346–53.

47. Masa JF, Celli BR, Riesco JA, et al. Noninvasive positive pressure ventilation and not oxygen may prevent overt ventilatory failure in patients with chest wall diseases. Chest 1997;112(1):207–13.

48. Borel J-C, Burel B, Tamisier R, et al. Comorbidities and mortality in hypercapnic obese under domiciliary noninvasive ventilation. PLoS One 2013;8(1):e52006.

49. Kushida CA, Chediak A, Berry RB, et al. Clinical guidelines for the manual titration of positive airway pressure in patients with obstructive sleep apnea. J Clin Sleep Med 2008;4(2):157–71.

50. BaHammam AS, Pandi-Perumal SR, Piper A, et al. Gender differences in patients with obesity hypoventilation syndrome. J Sleep Res 2016;25(4):445–53.

51. Manthous CA, Mokhlesi B. Avoiding management errors in patients with obesity hypoventilation syndrome. Ann Am Thorac Soc 2016;13(1):109–14.

# Noninvasive Mechanical Ventilation in Acute Ventilatory Failure
## Rationale and Current Applications

Antonio M. Esquinas, MD, PhD[a],*,
Maly Oron Benhamou, MD[b], Alastair J. Glossop, MD[c],
Bushra Mina, MD[b]

## KEYWORDS

- Noninvasive mechanical ventilation • Acute respiratory failure • Hypoxemic
- Chronic respiratory failure • COPD • Pneumonia • Cardiac pulmonary edema • Extubation

## KEY POINTS

- Noninvasive ventilation (NIV) plays a pivotal role in acute ventilator failure and has been shown, in certain disease processes such as acute exacerbation of chronic obstructive pulmonary disease, to prevent and shorten the duration of invasive mechanical ventilation, reducing the risks and complications associated with it.
- The application of NIV is relatively simple and well tolerated by patients and in the right setting can change the course of their illness.
- Appropriate indications, ventilatory equipment and ventilatory setting physicians training and patients selections are essentials.
- Early diagnosis and treatment of patient ventilator-asynchrony, evaluation of airflow, pressure volume and leaks monitoring are required.
- Still new emergent ventilatory modes, indications and prevention NIV failure need more large clinical trials.

## RATIONALE

Acute ventilatory failure in patients with severe hypercapnic and hypoxemic respiratory failure may require endotracheal intubation (ETI) and invasive mechanical ventilation (IMV).[1] In such patients, IMV is associated with significant morbidity and mortality.[2] The use of noninvasive ventilation (NIV) as an alternative to ETI in these circumstances reduces the incidence of serious complications and length of stay (LOS).[2,3] Over the last 15 years, NIV has become a widespread technique for ventilatory support in the intensive care unit (ICU). Currently, the main indications for treatment with NIV in the ICU include the following: acute exacerbation of chronic obstructive pulmonary disease (AECOPD), cardiogenic pulmonary edema (CPE), acute lung injury, community-acquired pneumonia, and postextubation respiratory failure as a means to avoid reintubation.[1]

[a] Intensive Care and Non-invasive Ventilatory Unit, Hospital Morales Meseguer, Avenida Marques Velez, Murcia 30008, Spain; [b] Department of Medicine, Division of Pulmonary and Critical Care Medicine, Northwell Health, Lenox Hill Hospital, New York, NY 10065, USA; [c] Department of Critical Care, Sheffield Teaching Hospitals NHS Foundation Trust, Royal Hallamshire Hospital, Glossop Road, Sheffield S10 2HE, UK
* Corresponding author.
E-mail address: antmesquinas@gmail.com

Sleep Med Clin 12 (2017) 597–606
http://dx.doi.org/10.1016/j.jsmc.2017.07.009

## PART 1. KEY PRACTICAL ASPECTS IN ACUTE VENTILATORY FAILURE: INTERFACE, DEVICES, AND PATIENT-VENTILATOR INTERACTION

### Interface

Facemasks (FM) are the gold-standard interface for NIV in acute respiratory failure (ARF). FMs are available in many different sizes and allow for ventilation through the nose and/or mouth.[4] Even though the quality, fit, and tolerability of FM have improved considerably, it is common to see nose bridge skin breakdown after a few days of use, necessitating the need for use of a different interface.[5] The experience with treatment of chronic respiratory failure or obstructive sleep apnea (OSA) provides other alternatives, such as nasal masks (NMs) and mouthpieces.[6] The use of NM for NIV in patients with ARF is limited, because these patients are usually "mouth breathers," resulting in major air leaks through the mouth, because the peak pressures are much higher than under nasal continuous positive airway pressure (CPAP). Another therapeutic option is the helmet, where there is no direct contact with the patient's face, and the occlusion is made at the level of neck.[7]

### Patient Ventilator Asynchrony

The characteristics (ie, dead space, compliance) of devices for bilevel positive airway pressure (BIPAP) have an important influence on patient-ventilator interaction.[8] A significant asynchrony between the beginning and the end of inspiratory support and the beginning and the end of patient inspiratory effort is commonly observed during BIPAP. Wasted efforts (when a patient's inspiratory effort was not followed by a ventilator cycle), auto-triggering (when a ventilator cycle occurs without being preceded by a patient's inspiratory effort), and prolonged inspirations (when each insufflation lasts longer than 1.5 seconds) may be also expected during NIV.[9] The patient-ventilator asynchrony is significantly higher during helmet BIPAP than during mask BIPAP.[8,9] Among the different masks, the asynchrony is more evident with mouthpiece compared with nasal or FM interfaces.[6] With regard to helmet use, the low elasticity and high inner volume of the device create a significant overdamping of pressure assistance and a deviation of ventilator-delivered flow from the patient in order to expand the compliant helmet (in particular, the soft collar) during BIPAP ventilation.[7] These impaired patient-ventilator interactions are responsible for the reduced efficiency of helmet BIPAP in unloading the respiratory muscles in conditions where increased respiratory muscle workload is a prominent feature.[10] A positive end-expiratory pressure (PEEP) of 6 cm $H_2O$ might be helpful in this clinical setting.[8,9] The use of higher flows and higher pressures, if tolerated by patients, may also reduce the compliance of the helmet and optimize the efficiency of helmet BIPAP.[10]

## PART 2. CURRENT INDICATIONS

### Acute on Chronic Hypercapnic Respiratory Failure

Hypercapnia is defined as the elevation of the arterial partial pressure of $CO_2$ ($Pa_{CO_2}$) >45 mm Hg, often as a result of either an increase in the dead space or decrease in the alveolar ventilation.[11] Hypercapnic respiratory failure may arise as a result of many causes and can be acute or acute on chronic, for example, in AECOPD or neuromuscular disorders at a time of acute illness (fever, infection, and so forth).[12] NIV has been extensively studied in the setting of hypercapnic respiratory failure and is considered the benchmark of treatment of AECOPD. During an AECOPD, the application of IPAP has been shown to subsequently result in a decrease in $Pa_{CO_2}$, increase in the partial pressure of arterial oxygen ($Pa_{O_2}$), increase in pH, decrease in work of breathing (WOB), increase in tidal volume, and, as a result, a decrease in respiratory rate.[13,14]

When comparing outcomes of patients treated with NIV with those who received IMV at time of admission for AECOPD, patients treated with NIV had lower inpatient mortality, shorter LOS, and reduced incidence of nosocomial pneumonia.[15] A large prospective study looking at ICU admissions with severe AECOPD found that those initially treated with NIV had a 61% lower risk of dying in the ICU, a shorter ICU stay, and a 41% lower risk of hospital mortality when compared with those who were initially treated with ETI after matching for severity of illness.[16] These benefits are likely to be at least partially attributable to the avoidance of complications associated with IMV, such as ventilator-associated pneumonia and barotrauma. On the other hand, patients who failed NIV (defined as a later need for IMV) had the highest mortality and a longer hospital stay when compared with those who initially received IMV.[16] A Simplified Acute Physiology Score (SAPS II) greater than 34 was reported to be independently associated with need for IMV,[17] and the likelihood of NIV failure increases sharply with higher SAPS II scores.[16,17]

### Obesity Hypoventilation Syndrome

Obesity hypoventilation syndrome (OHS) is defined as an awake $Pa_{CO_2}$ >45 mm Hg in an individual with a body mass index >30 kg/m$^2$ when other causes of chronic alveolar hypoventilation have been ruled out. Serum bicarbonate level (>27 mmol/L) in the absence of another cause for a metabolic alkalosis may be included in the definition of OHS.[18,19] These populations are characterized by marked decrease in lung volumes, impaired respiratory muscle performance, restricted diaphragmatic excursion, and greater reductions in respiratory system compliance compared with those with eucapnic obesity.[19] These factors all contribute to the increased WOB at rest. Blunted ventilatory responsiveness to hypoxia and hypercapnia is also frequently seen. In patients with OHS, NIV therapy remains the mainstay of treatment and reverses daytime respiratory failure in 50% to 80% of patients.[20] It is effective in controlling sleep-disordered breathing associated with the syndrome, maintaining airway patency, increasing functional residual capacity, decreasing WOB, and improving awake blood gases in most individuals.[21] Patients with OHS may also benefit from NIV application during episodes of ARF. Patients with OHS have an increased WOB even during quiet breathing, with a direct correlation to $Paco_2$ levels,[20,21] which results in a decreased ventilatory reserve during an acute event such as infection.[22] Early application of NIV, especially BIPAP, has been shown to result in a reduced requirement for IMV by increasing alveolar ventilation as well as maintaining upper airway patency.[19–21] The incidence of postoperative complications is higher among OHS patients undergoing elective noncardiac surgery and often is unrecognized at the time of surgery.[23,24] Hypercapnic-OHS patients are more prone to postoperative respiratory failure (odds ratio [OR], 10.9; 95% confidence interval [CI], 3.7–32.3; $P<.0001$), postoperative heart failure (OR, 5.4; 95% CI, 1.9–15.7; $P = .002$), prolonged intubation (OR, 3.1; 95% CI, 0.6–15.3; $P = .2$), postoperative ICU transfer (OR, 10.9; 95% CI, 3.7–32.3; $P<.0001$), and longer ICU ($\beta$-coefficient, 0.86; standard error [SE], 0.32; $P = .009$) and hospital ($\beta$-coefficient, 2.94; SE, 0.87; $P = .0008$) LOSs when compared with normocapnic OSA patients. NIV may have a critical role in preventing and reversing postoperative complications associated with OHS.[24,25]

## Neuromuscular Disorders

NIV also has an important role in the acute treatment of patients with *neuromuscular disorders*. In a patient cohort with an already limited ventilator reserve, muscle weakness results in increased thoracic restriction, and thus, atelectasis and alveolar hypoventilation.[26–28] When treating patients with neuromuscular disorders, timing is crucial to the success rate of NIV.[26,28] Once severe fatigue and hypercapnia develop, patients are more likely to fail NIV, with the presence of paradoxic breathing being the most reliable sign for impending ARF.[27]

Another consideration when planning NIV therapy is the presence of bulbar muscular weakness, seen more commonly in patients with Guillain-Barré, myasthenia gravis, or amyotrophic lateral sclerosis. This may not only result in upper airway obstruction but also place patients who are unable to handle their secretions at an elevated risk of aspiration.[29] The use of BIPAP in this group is preferred because it also provides support for the respiratory muscles.[30] In patients with a myasthenic crisis, the use of BIPAP may prevent the need for ETI and shorten the time needed for ventilation as well as the length of ICU and hospital stay.[31]

## Acute Cardiogenic Pulmonary Edema

Positive pressure ventilation has well-established effects on the pathophysiology of pulmonary edema.[32,33] It enables recovery of respiratory function by improving pulmonary compliance and shunt as well as off-loading the respiratory muscles.[33,34] Most studies examining the use of NIV in acute cardiogenic pulmonary edema (ACPE) have been conducted within ICU, but it is important to consider that NIV, unlike mechanical ventilation, is an intervention that may be used to deliver ventilatory support outside of critical care units in the treatment of ACPE. *NIV-CPAP* may reverse the pathologic changes that occur during ACPE via recruitment of flooded alveoli, increasing functional residual capacity, and counterbalancing any intrinsic positive PEEP; respiratory system compliance is increased as a net effect. With regard to hemodynamics, PEEP improves oxygenation through a reduction of both shunt and afterload by increasing ventricular transmural pressure. This mechanical effect is of great clinical significance, because the respiratory distress encountered in ACPE is not directly related to hypoxemia and therefore cannot be reversed with oxygen therapy alone.[35,36]

### Noninvasive ventilation–bilevel positive airway pressure
Although CPAP helps restoration of the normal physiologic respiratory pattern, BIPAP offers a greater mechanical support to respiratory muscle when exhaustion is becoming severe.[36]

### Continuous positive airway pressure vs bilevel positive airway pressure
In a recent systemic review, Pang and colleagues[37] concluded that CPAP in ACPE is associated with a decrease in ETI rate and a trend to a decrease in hospital mortality when compared with standard therapy alone, that is, high-flow oxygen. These results have been recently confirmed by Masip,[38] who demonstrated that CPAP and

BIPAP decreased mortality during ACPE by 47% and 40%, respectively, when compared with standard therapy. Several uncontrolled trials support the theory that BIPAP is an effective treatment of ACPE by demonstrating low ETI and low complication rates. These results strongly support the advice of Wysocki and Antonelli[39] that any form of NIV, either CPAP or BIPAP, may be effective in preventing ETI in ACPE.

Several trials have demonstrated that patients with ACPE are frequently hypercapnic, at least partly as a result of respiratory muscle fatigue and inability to maintain adequate ventilation. CPAP is able to improve the WOB, but unloading of respiratory muscles may be best achieved by BIPAP. In general, there is a significant improvement in several important respiratory and hemodynamic parameters in patients with ACPE receiving BIPAP, whereas patients in the CPAP group only showed significant improvement in respiratory rate.[40]

### Blunt Chest Trauma

Systematic review analysis determinates controversial use of NIV in chest trauma.[41,42] Noninvasive CPAP with PCA led to lower mortality and nosocomial infection rates. Oxygenation and length of ICU stay were similar. The findings suggest that CPAP should be trialed as the initial supportive treatment of flail chest caused by blunt thoracic trauma.[41,42]

### Immunosuppression (Hematologic and Solid Malignancies)

Prognosis of hematologic malignancy has significantly improved over the last 2 decades because of advances in diagnosis as well as therapy.[43,44] NIV has been suggested as an important alternative to conventional IMV in this patient population as a means to avoid complications related to ETI. Hilbert and colleagues[45] randomized 52 immunosuppressed patients who developed acute hypoxemic respiratory failure because of pulmonary disease to receive NIV or standard treatment, consisting of delivering a high fraction of inspired oxygen through a facial mask. In the NIV group, ETI could be averted in 14 (54%) cases compared with 6 (23%) cases in the standard treatment group. ICU and in-hospital mortality were 38% and 50% versus 69% and 81%, respectively. Azoulay and colleagues conducted a multicenter study looking at factors related to outcome in patients with ARF with cancer. The benefits of NIV versus IMV as a means to treat ARF in these patients are more subtle.[46] As the data by Hilbert and colleagues[45] show, an NIV trial can be considered in an early phase of ARF as a prophylactic measure to halt or slow further respiratory deterioration, while the underlying disease is searched for and treated aggressively. Thus, by avoiding ETI and related complications, NIV can reduce intubation-attributable mortality in a selected group of patients.[43,44] However, when patients are admitted to the ICU in a more advanced state of ARF, this protective effect of NIV seems to be lost.[44,46]

### The Use of Noninvasive Ventilation in Weaning from Invasive Mechanical Ventilation

NIV has been studied as an alternative to IMV in patients who are weaning from IMV but have failed a spontaneous breathing trial and thus are not deemed suitable for extubation.[47,48] Extubation of such patients onto NIV provides continued ventilatory support without the damaging effects of ongoing IMV and sedation[49]; a degree of contention over the use of NIV in this setting remains because of conflicting results and uncertainty regarding optimal patient selection. After several smaller studies had demonstrated benefits from using NIV in weaning patients from IMV,[50,51] a *Cochrane Review* studying the use of NIV to wean patients versus continued IMV weaning was published.[49,52] The investigators concluded that reduced ICU and hospital LOS, rates of ventilator associated pneumonia (VAP), as well as decrease in mortality were seen with NIV weaning, in particular patients with chronic obstructive pulmonary disease (COPD).

### Use of Noninvasive Ventilation After Extubation

Reported rates of extubation failure, defined as the need for reintubation within 48 to 72 hours of extubation, vary greatly in the literature but may be as high as 19% in some series.[53,54] Failed extubation is a highly significant event for many patients, with an increased morbidity and mortality seen, and thus NIV may have an important role to play in the prevention of these sequelae.[55]

#### Prevention of after-extubation respiratory failure

Several studies have used NIV after extubation as a preventative strategy in patients identified as being high risk for extubation failure before cessation of IMV.[49,52] When used in this manner, "prophylactic" NIV has been demonstrated to reduce reintubation rates, incidence of VAP, and mortality. It has also been suggested from the evidence that NIV used prophylactically after extubation in morbidly obese patients, an increasing problem encountered in Critical Care units worldwide, may reduce rates of reintubation.[52]

## Treatment of after-extubation respiratory failure

NIV has also been used to treat respiratory distress that may develop after extubation and result in reinstitution of IMV.[47] Studies in this area have provided less compelling results to support NIV use.[56] A landmark study by Esteban and colleagues[56] found that NIV use in patients with after-extubation respiratory distress led to an increased mortality compared with standard medical therapy. It is of note that the NIV group received much longer periods of ineffective NIV before reintubation (13 vs 4 hours on average), which may have contributed to the excess mortality. Subgroup analysis suggested some benefit for NIV when used in patients with known COPD.

A subsequent meta-analysis of 10 trials of after-extubation NIV use pooled data from 1382 patients and grouped studies into "prophylaxis" and "treatment" groups. The investigators concluded that significant patient benefits were seen with NIV prophylaxis but not treatment of after-extubation respiratory failure, thus supporting the findings of earlier work.[49,52]

It is evident that patient selection is paramount in the success of NIV after extubation, along with timing and duration of intervention. Debate also surrounds the definition of "high risk" of extubation failure and which strategies should be used in lower-risk populations. Recent work by Thille and colleagues demonstrated a significantly reduced risk of "high-risk" patients requiring reintubation within 7 days of being extubated with prophylactic NIV use. Of note, NIV was used early and for prolonged periods of time in this study, and more than 60% of patients screened met the criteria for being high risk.

NIV has a very important role to play in both weaning from IMV and also prevention of after-extubation respiratory failure in selected patient groups. This is reflected in recent guidelines issued by the British Thoracic Society, which recommends use of NIV to aid weaning of patients with COPD and prevention of extubation failure in high-risk patients.[57]

## The Use of Noninvasive Ventilation in Postoperative Patients

The respiratory system is subject to several major physiologic changes during surgery and general anesthesia, and many of these changes incline patients toward the development of postoperative respiratory failure. Postoperative pulmonary complications (PPCs) have an overall incidence of 5% to 10% in European surgical cohorts, but may be as high as 40% following surgical procedures that involve breach of the abdominal and thoracic cavities.

NIV is an attractive therapy in postoperative patients because the alveolar recruitment, improved oxygenation, and reduced WOB seen with NIV may directly attenuate the problems created by major surgery that predispose patients to the development of PPC.[24,25,58]

## Prophylactic postoperative noninvasive ventilation

NIV has been studied as a prophylactic intervention in patients deemed to be at increased risk of developing PPC following major surgery in several specific surgical fields.[59] Use of CPAP prophylactically following major abdominal surgery has been demonstrated to reduce rates of pneumonia, reintubation, and critical care LOS in a large randomized controlled trial. These findings were replicated in a meta-analysis of NIV use following abdominal surgery by the Cochrane group.[58] CPAP has also been demonstrated to improve oxygenation and reduce the incidence of PPC following thoracic and abdominal vascular surgical procedures, and also after cardiac surgery when applied prophylactically for the first 24 hours postoperatively.[59–61] However, despite robust evidence from well-conducted studies to support prophylactic use of NIV postoperatively, barriers to more widespread implementation are often encountered, frequently because of patient discomfort and lack of compliance.

## Therapeutic postoperative noninvasive ventilation

Development of respiratory failure that requires reintubation is associated with a significant increase in mortality following high-risk surgical procedures such as esophageal and lung resection surgery, where reintubation may confer mortality as high as 60% to 80%.[62] The application of NIV to avert the need for IMV in these postoperative groups is therefore an important therapeutic option. In a landmark study by Auriant and colleagues,[63] mortality in patients developing respiratory failure following lung resection surgery was significantly reduced from 37.5% to 12.5% with the use of BIPAP. Application of BIPAP to patients developing respiratory failure following esophageal surgery was also demonstrated to reduce rates of reintubation and critical care LOS.[64] It is also of note that in both of these studies, no increase in surgical anastomosis failure was reported with NIV use.

Benefits from NIV use have also been reported following several other procedures, including Transplant and Bariatric surgery, and also in specific groups of patients, including the obese and patients with sleep apnea in the perioperative period.[65]

Most studies published on the postoperative use of NIV report beneficial effects on patient outcomes, although only a very small number actually impact mortality. It must, however, be remembered that baseline mortality from elective surgical procedures is very low, even for high-risk procedures, and thus the ability of any single intervention to impact this will be limited.

## Unconventional and Emergent Noninvasive Ventilation Applications

NIV may be a beneficial supportive intervention in a range of upper airway and gastrointestinal endoscopy procedures.[66] Such procedures pose many challenges in the management of patients, especially those at high risk of respiratory failure, because the administration of sedation may result in respiratory depression, loss of upper airway patency, and aspiration.[67] Ventilation may also be compromised during tracheal and bronchoscopic procedures by the presence of the endoscopic probe in the patient airway. Cabrini and colleagues[68] performed a systematic review of studies using NIV during a variety of upper airway and gastrointestinal endoscopies (including bronchoscopy, fiberoptic bronchoscopy–guided tracheal intubation, placement of percutaneous endoscopic gastrostomy, gastroscopy, transesophageal echocardiography). They demonstrated high success rates with NIV use, even in patients who were at high risk of respiratory failure, such as hypoxemic or sedated patients. This benefit was pronounced in those undergoing bronchoscopy with or without bronchoalveolar lavage as a means to avoid periprocedural hypoxemia.[68]

NIV has also been studied as an aid to preoxygenation before ETI and has been demonstrated to result in fewer desaturations when compared with the traditional bag-mask ventilation technique.[69]

## PART 3. NONINVASIVE VENTILATION: RESPONSE AND COMPLICATIONS
### Noninvasive Ventilation Failure

NIV failure is defined as the need to withdraw the therapy for subsequent ETI or a movement to a more palliative strategy.[17,70,71] Failure may be early (up to 24 hours after initiation of NIV) or late (more than 48 hours). The causes of early failure have been extensively studied, whereas the causes of late failure remain less well understood.

### Hypercapnic noninvasive ventilation failure
Moretti and colleagues[71] showed that the rate of NIV failure in COPD with ARF ranges from 5% to 40%, with many of the studies reporting an

incidence of late failure of around 10% to 20%. Early identification of patients who may be categorized into this subset is critical to avoid undue delay in ETI.

**Identification of risk factors for noninvasive ventilation failure** There are several readily identifiable patient comorbidities and pathophysiologic characteristics that may predict a poor response to NIV trials, such as follows: *Age:* In general, ARF carries a poor prognosis among patients of advanced age and poor functional status. *Comorbidity:* A critical factor related to deterioration in the progression of these patients, comorbidity is particularly correlated with diabetes and chronic renal failure. *Severity:* Several studies have suggested that higher severity of illness scores (measured with APACHE II and SAPS II severity scales) are correlated with a very poor prognosis in patients with ARF treated with NIV. *Type of ARF:* A higher incidence of failure of NIV is seen among patients with ARF secondary to non–rapidly reversible diseases, such as pneumonia, myocardial infarction, and sepsis. *Hypercapnia:* The efficacy of NIV in hypercapnic respiratory failure with moderate acidemia has been demonstrated in numerous studies. However, severe acidemia (pH <7.2) related to very high $CO_2$ levels is a strong predictor of poor outcomes with NIV treatment, especially if the pH fails to correct with NIV therapy.[72,73]

### Hypoxemic noninvasive ventilation failure
Hypoxemia is a key determinant factor in the failure or success of NIV in patients with ARF. It is important to consider the cause of respiratory failure (cardiogenic or noncardiogenic), the degree of severity of hypoxemia, and also the response to NIV.[17] Measures to recruit the alveolar units and unload the respiratory muscles should be optimized to enhance the likelihood of success of NIV in hypoxemic patients. Factors recognized to contribute to the failure of NIV in treating hypoxemic ARF include the following.

**Persistent muscular fatigue** Respiratory muscles have a limited capacity to maintain gas exchange in the face of structural injury or functional deterioration, and persistent fatigue is frequently associated with late NIV failure. Its presence is also a poor prognostic indicator in patients undergoing treatment with NIV for hypoxemic ARF.

**Persistent dyspnea** Failure of NIV to improve dyspnea is a predictor of treatment failure. Control of dyspnea is critical in this patient group, and in some circumstances, pharmacologic agents that decrease the threshold of dyspnea perception (such as opiate and anxiolytic medications) should be considered.

**Level of consciousness** A low level of consciousness (Glasgow Coma Scale [GCS] <9) is frequently quoted as an indication for ETI to provide airway protection and to reduce the risk of pulmonary aspiration. Several studies have highlighted the utility of NIV in patients with a GCS less than 9, usually as a result of hypercapnia in COPD. A lack of clinical and blood gas improvement during the first hour of treatment is a predictor of NIV failure.

## Interface failure and patient-ventilator asynchrony

The problems encountered with interfaces and patient-ventilator asynchrony when treating ARF with NIV may frequently lead to suboptimal delivery of ventilator support and increase the likelihood of treatment failure.[4,8,10,72] Several interlinking factors may contribute to this, including the following: *Interface selection:* One of the main causes of NIV failure lies with the technical inconveniences of an FM, notably incorrect size and inadequate seal. *Leaks:* Values below the double of patient's minute volume are tolerated, although above this level the efficacy of treatment is greatly reduced. *Pressure ulceration:* One of the most frequently reported and well-described complications of treatment with NIV is the pressure ulcer. Advances in interface design, technical improvements in the quality of interfaces, and also adoption of a "rotating interface" policy may all help to reduce the incidence of pressure ulceration secondary to NIV treatment. *Mask:* Evidence from several studies has suggested that the type of mask is more important than the ventilation mode applied to the success of NIV in patients with hypercapnic respiratory failure. NMs are often better tolerated, although less effective, than full FMs. Recently, a new type of mask has been developed, the "helmet" mask, which has been effective in decreasing ETI rates and mask-related complications when compared with more traditional interfaces. Despite these advances, however, mask intolerance remains a major factor in NIV treatment failure.

In summary, NIV treatment efficiency should be controlled by closely monitoring clinical signs (eg, comfort, dyspnea, respiratory frequency, symptoms of accessory muscle work) as well as biochemical markers such as pH, $Pao_2$, and $Paco_2$ levels. It is also vital that close attention is paid to the degree of interface displacement, patient tolerance of therapy, and degree of patient-mask-ventilator adaptation to ensure optimal delivery of ventilator support and reduce the risks of treatment failure.

## Complications

NIV as a treatment modality for ARF arguably confers the advantage of being associated with fewer and less severe complications, when compared with those associated with IMV.[5] However, it must be remembered that NIV retains a failure rate that will necessitate progression onto requiring IMV and still provides several notable challenges and complications when used to treat ARF. The most frequent complications associated with NIV include the following[5,74]: *Discomfort:* Discomfort is frequently reported by patients and represents an unpleasant sensation that is related to the device or pressure values adopted during BIPAP delivery. *Claustrophobia:* Claustrophobia is a frequently reported sensation by patients receiving NIV via tight-fitting interfaces. *Nasal bridge problems:* Nasal pain, either mucosal or on the bridge of the nose, and nasal bridge erythema or ulceration from mask pressure account for a large portion of reported complications of mask BIPAP. *Nasal or oral dryness and nasal congestion:* Nasal or oral dryness is often reported by patients receiving treatment with NIV and is the result of high airflow, air leaking through the patient's mouth during treatment, and inadequate humidification of inspired gases. *Aspiration pneumonia:* Aspiration pneumonia has been reported in up to 5% of patients receiving treatment with NIV and may arise because of the presence of raised gastric pressures in a patient with an unprotected airway. *Gastric distention:* Gastric insufflation is reported in up to 50% of patients receiving BIPAP but is rarely intolerable and is usually adequately managed by placement of a nasogastric tube. *Barotrauma:* Barotrauma is a well-recognized complication of positive pressure ventilation. It is a pulmonary injury resulting from alveolar overdistention and can lead to pulmonary interstitial emphysema, pneumomediastinum, subcutaneous emphysema, and pneumothorax. *Hemodynamic effects:* In general, BIPAP is well tolerated hemodynamically, presumably because of the low inflation pressures used compared with invasive ventilation. In the short term, use of BIPAP may result in a reduced heart rate, systolic blood pressure, and systemic vascular resistance. In patients receiving optimal therapy, the reduction of systolic blood pressure is rarely significant and may actually be associated with an increase in ejection fraction and cardiac output.

## SUMMARY

NIV plays a pivotal role in acute ventilator failure and has been shown, in certain disease processes such as AECOPD, to prevent and shorten the duration of IMV, reducing the risks and complications associated with it. The application of NIV is relatively simple and well tolerated by patients, and in the right setting, can change the course of their illness.

## REFERENCES

1. Bello G, De Pascale G, Antonelli M. Noninvasive ventilation. Clin Chest Med 2016;37(4):711–21.
2. Brochard L. Mechanical ventilation: invasive versus noninvasive. Eur Respir J Suppl 2003;47:31s–7s.
3. Crimi C, Noto A, Princi P, et al. European survey of noninvasive ventilation practices. Eur Respir J 2010;36(2):362–9.
4. Pisani L, Carlucci A, Nava S. Interfaces for noninvasive mechanical ventilation: technical aspects and efficiency. Minerva Anestesiol 2012;78(10):1154–61.
5. Carron M, Freo U, BaHammam AS, et al. Complications of non-invasive ventilation techniques: a comprehensive qualitative review of randomized trials. Br J Anaesth 2013;110(6):896–914.
6. Pinto T, Chatwin M, Banfi P, et al. Mouthpiece ventilation and complementary techniques in patients with neuromuscular disease: a brief clinical review and update. Chron Respir Dis 2017;14(2):187–93.
7. Esquinas AM, Consentini R, Pravinkumar E, et al. Effectiveness of helmet non-invasive ventilation with external PEEP valves: key remains inside the helmet. Minerva Anestesiol 2013;79(6):697–8.
8. Hess DR. Patient-ventilator interaction during noninvasive ventilation. Respir Care 2011;56(2):153–65.
9. Scala R, Naldi M. Ventilators for noninvasive ventilation to treat acute respiratory failure. Respir Care 2008;53(8):1054–80.
10. Vignaux L, Tassaux D, Jolliet P. Performance of noninvasive ventilation modes on ICU ventilators during pressure support: a bench model study. Intensive Care Med 2007;33(8):1444–51.
11. Ambrosino N, Vagheggini G. Noninvasive positive pressure ventilation in the acute care setting: where are we? Eur Respir J 2008;31(4):874–86.
12. Song Y, Chen R, Zhan Q, et al. The optimum timing to wean invasive ventilation for patients with AECOPD or COPD with pulmonary infection. Int J Chron Obstruct Pulmon Dis 2016;11:535–42.
13. Ramsay M, Hart N. Current opinions on non-invasive ventilation as a treatment for chronic obstructive pulmonary disease. Curr Opin Pulm Med 2013;19(6):626–30.
14. Brochard L, Mancebo J, Elliott MW. Noninvasive ventilation for acute respiratory failure. Eur Respir J 2002;19(4):712–21.
15. Lindenauer PK, Stefan MS, Shieh MS, et al. Outcomes associated with invasive and noninvasive ventilation among patients hospitalized with exacerbations of chronic obstructive pulmonary disease. JAMA Intern Med 2014;174(12):1982–93.
16. Stefan MS, Nathanson BH, Priya A, et al. Hospitals' patterns of use of noninvasive ventilation in patients with asthma exacerbation. Chest 2016;149(3):729–36.
17. Antonelli M, Conti G, Moro ML, et al. Predictors of failure of noninvasive positive pressure ventilation in patients with acute hypoxemic respiratory failure: a multi-center study. Intensive Care Med 2001;27(11):1718–28.
18. Sequeira TC, BaHammam AS, Esquinas AM. Noninvasive ventilation in the critically ill patient with obesity hypoventilation syndrome: a review. J Intensive Care Med 2017;32(7):421–8.
19. Pépin JL, Timsit JF, Tamisier R, et al. Prevention and care of respiratory failure in obese patients. Lancet Respir Med 2016;4(5):407–18.
20. Jones SF, Brito V, Ghamande S. Obesity hypoventilation syndrome in the critically ill. Crit Care Clin 2015;31(3):419–34.
21. Nicolini A, Banfi P, Grecchi B, et al. Non-invasive ventilation in the treatment of sleep-related breathing disorders: a review and update. Rev Port Pneumol 2014;20(6):324–35.
22. Kress JP, Pohlman AS, Alverdy J, et al. The impact of morbid obesity on oxygen cost of breathing (VO(2RESP)) at rest. Am J Respir Crit Care Med 1999;160(3):883–6.
23. Carron M, Zarantonello F, Tellaroli P, et al. Perioperative noninvasive ventilation in obese patients: a qualitative review and meta-analysis. Surg Obes Relat Dis 2016;12(3):681–91.
24. Jaber S, De Jong A, Castagnoli A, et al. Non-invasive ventilation after surgery. Ann Fr Anesth Reanim 2014;33(7–8):487–91.
25. Jaber S, Michelet P, Chanques G. Role of non-invasive ventilation (NIV) in the perioperative period. Best Pract Res Clin Anaesthesiol 2010;24(2):253–65.
26. Vianello A, Bevilacqua M, Arcaro G, et al. Non-invasive ventilatory approach to treatment of acute respiratory failure in neuromuscular disorders. A comparison with endotracheal intubation. Intensive Care Med 2000;26(4):384–90.
27. Rabinstein AA. Acute neuromuscular respiratory failure. Continuum (Minneap Minn) 2015;21(5 Neurocritical Care):1324–45.
28. Bach JR, Gonçalves MR, Hon A, et al. Changing trends in the management of end-stage neuromuscular respiratory muscle failure: recommendations

of an international consensus. Am J Phys Med Rehabil 2013;92(3):267–77.

29. Rabinstein AA. Noninvasive ventilation for neuro-muscular respiratory failure: when to use and when to avoid. Curr Opin Crit Care 2016;22(2):94–9.

30. Gregoretti C, Pisani L, Cortegiani A, et al. Noninvasive ventilation in critically ill patients. Crit Care Clin 2015;31(3):435–57.

31. Seneviratne J, Mandrekar J, Wijdicks EF, et al. Noninvasive ventilation in myasthenic crisis. Arch Neurol 2008;65(1):54–8.

32. Cotter G, Kaluski E, Moshkovitz Y, et al. Pulmonary edema: new insight on pathogenesis and treatment. Curr Opin Cardiol 2001;16(3):159–63.

33. Gray A, Goodacre S, Newby DE, et al, 3CPO Trialists. Noninvasive ventilation in acute cardiogenic pulmonary edema. N Engl J Med 2008;359(2):142–51.

34. Nava S, Carbone G, DiBattista N, et al. Noninvasive ventilation in cardiogenic pulmonary edema: a multicenter randomized trial. Am J Respir Crit Care Med 2003;168(12):1432–7.

35. Nouira S, Boukef R, Bouida W, et al. Non-invasive pressure support ventilation and CPAP in cardiogenic pulmonary edema: a multicenter randomized study in the emergency department. Intensive Care Med 2011;37(2):249–56.

36. Vital FM, Saconato H, Ladeira MT, et al. Non-invasive positive pressure ventilation (CPAP or bilevel NPPV) for cardiogenic pulmonary edema. Cochrane Database Syst Rev 2008;(3):CD005351.

37. Pang D, Keenan SP, Cook DJ, et al. The effect of positive pressure airway support on mortality and the need for intubation in cardiogenic pulmonary edema: a systematic review. Chest 1998;114(4): 1185–92.

38. Masip J. Noninvasive ventilation in acute cardiogenic pulmonary edema. Curr Opin Crit Care 2008;14(5):531–5.

39. Wysocki M, Antonelli M. Noninvasive mechanical ventilation in acute hypoxaemic respiratory failure. Eur Respir J 2001;18(1):209–20.

40. Weng CL, Zhao YT, Liu QH, et al. Meta-analysis: noninvasive ventilation in acute cardiogenic pulmonary edema. Ann Intern Med 2010;152(9):590–600.

41. Chiumello D, Coppola S, Froio S, et al. Noninvasive ventilation in chest trauma: systematic review and meta-analysis. Intensive Care Med 2013;39(7): 1171–80.

42. Duggal A, Perez P, Golan E, et al. Safety and efficacy of noninvasive ventilation in patients with blunt chest trauma: a systematic review. Crit Care 2013; 17(4):R142.

43. Saillard C, Mokart D, Lemiale V, et al. Mechanical ventilation in cancer patients. Minerva Anestesiol 2014;80(6):712–25.

44. Bello G, De Pascale G, Antonelli M. Noninvasive ventilation for the immunocompromised patient: always appropriate? Curr Opin Crit Care 2012; 18(1):54–60.

45. Hilbert G, Gruson D, Vargas F, et al. Noninvasive ventilation in immunosuppressed patients with pulmonary infiltrates, fever, and acute respiratory failure. N Engl J Med 2001;344(7):481–7.

46. Lemiale V, Resche-Rigon M, Mokart D, et al. Acute respiratory failure in patients with hematological malignancies: outcomes according to initial ventilation strategy. A groupe de recherche respiratoire en réanimation onco-hématologique (Grrr-OH) study. Ann Intensive Care 2015;5(1):28.

47. Rose L. Strategies for weaning from mechanical ventilation: a state of the art review. Intensive Crit Care Nurs 2015;31(4):189–95.

48. Ambrosino N, Gabbrielli L. The difficult-to-wean patient. Expert Rev Respir Med 2010;4(5):685–92.

49. Glossop AJ, Shephard N, Bryden DC, et al. Non-invasive ventilation for weaning, avoiding reintubation after extubation and in the postoperative period: a meta-analysis. Br J Anaesth 2012; 109(3):305–14.

50. Ferrer M, Esquinas A, Arancibia F, et al. Noninvasive ventilation during persistent weaning failure: a randomized controlled trial. Am J Respir Crit Care Med 2003;168(1):70–6.

51. Esquinas AM, Glossop A. Noninvasive ventilation strategy for weaning from mechanical ventilation for underlying COPD: how to get to be great being little? Lung India 2015;32(1):90–1.

52. Burns KE, Adhikari NK, Keenan SP, et al. Noninvasive positive pressure ventilation as a weaning strategy for intubated adults with respiratory failure. Cochrane Database Syst Rev 2010;(8):CD004127.

53. Krishna B, Sampath S, Moran JL. The role of non-invasive positive pressure ventilation in post-extubation respiratory failure: an evaluation using meta-analytic techniques. Indian J Crit Care Med 2013;17(4):253–61.

54. Lin C, Yu H, Fan H, et al. The efficacy of noninvasive ventilation in managing postextubation respiratory failure: a meta-analysis. Heart Lung 2014; 43(2):99–104.

55. Ornico SR, Lobo SM, Sanches HS, et al. Noninvasive ventilation immediately after extubation improves weaning outcome after acute respiratory failure: a randomized controlled trial. Crit Care 2013;17(2):R39.

56. Esteban A, Frutos-Vivar F, Ferguson ND, et al. Noninvasive positive-pressure ventilation for respiratory failure after extubation. N Engl J Med 2004; 350(24):2452–60.

57. Schmidt GA, Girard TD, Kress JP, et al, ATS/CHEST Ad Hoc Committee on Liberation from Mechanical Ventilation in Adults. Official executive summary of an American Thoracic Society/American College of Chest Physicians clinical practice guideline:

liberation from mechanical ventilation in critically ill adults. Am J Respir Crit Care Med 2016;195(1): 115–9.

58. Ireland CJ, Chapman TM, Mathew SF, et al. Continuous positive airway pressure (CPAP) during the postoperative period for prevention of postoperative morbidity and mortality following major abdominal surgery. Cochrane Database Syst Rev 2014;(8): CD008930.

59. Chiumello D, Chevallard G, Gregoretti C. Non-invasive ventilation in postoperative patients: a systematic review. Intensive Care Med 2011;37(6):918–29.

60. Landoni G, Zangrillo A, Cabrini L. Noninvasive ventilation after cardiac and thoracic surgery in adult patients: a review. J Cardiothorac Vasc Anesth 2012; 26(5):917–22.

61. Guarracino F, Ambrosino N. Non invasive ventilation in cardio-surgical patients. Minerva Anestesiol 2011; 77(7):734–41.

62. Torres MF, Porfirio GJ, Carvalho AP, et al. Non-invasive positive pressure ventilation for prevention of complications after pulmonary resection in lung cancer patients. Cochrane Database Syst Rev 2015;(9): CD010355.

63. Auriant I, Jallot A, Hervé P, et al. Noninvasive ventilation reduces mortality in acute respiratory failure following lung resection. Am J Respir Crit Care Med 2001;164(7):1231–5.

64. Michelet P, D'Journo XB, Seinaye F, et al. Non-invasive ventilation for treatment of postoperative respiratory failure alter oesophagectomy. Br J Surg 2009;96(1):54–60.

65. Hu XY. Effective ventilation strategies for obese patients undergoing bariatric surgery: a literature review. AANA J 2016;84(1):35–45.

66. Ambrosino N, Guarracino F. Unusual applications of noninvasive ventilation. Eur Respir J 2011;38(2): 440–9.

67. Hilbert G, Clouzeau B, Nam Bui H, et al. Sedation during non-invasive ventilation. Minerva Anestesiol 2012;78(7):842–6.

68. Cabrini L, Nobile L, Cama E, et al. Non-invasive ventilation during upper endoscopies in adult patients. A systematic review. Minerva Anestesiol 2013;79(6):683–94.

69. Baillard C, Fosse JP, Sebbane M, et al. Noninvasive ventilation improves preoxygenation before intubation of hypoxic patients. Am J Respir Crit Care Med 2006;174(2):171–7.

70. Martín-González F, González-Robledo J, Sánchez-Hernández F, et al. Success/failure prediction of noninvasive mechanical ventilation in intensive care units. Using multiclassifiers and feature selection methods. Methods Inf Med 2016;55(3):234–41.

71. Moretti M, Cilione C, Tampieri A, et al. Incidence and causes of non-invasive mechanical ventilation failure after initial success. Thorax 2000;55(10):819–25.

72. Ozyilmaz E, Ugurlu AO, Nava S. Timing of noninvasive ventilation failure: causes, risk factors, and potential remedies. BMC Pulm Med 2014;14:19.

73. Phua J, Kong K, Lee KH, et al. Noninvasive ventilation in hypercapnic acute respiratory failure due to chronic obstructive pulmonary disease vs. other conditions: effectiveness and predictors of failure. Intensive Care Med 2005;31(4):533–9.

74. Raurell-Torredà M, Argilaga-Molero E, Colomer-Plana M, et al. Optimising non-invasive mechanical ventilation: which unit should care for these patients? A cohort study. Aust Crit Care 2016;30(4): 225–33.

# Noninvasive Positive Pressure Ventilatory Support Begins During Sleep

CrossMark

John R. Bach, MD[a,b],*

## KEYWORDS

- Noninvasive ventilation • Noninvasive ventilatory support
- Continuous noninvasive intermittent positive pressure ventilatory support
- Continuous positive airway pressure • Mechanical insufflation-exsufflation • Ventilatory pump failure
- Neuromuscular disease

## KEY POINTS

- Patients with weak or paralyzed respiratory muscles should only be prescribed and use sleep nasal NVS when symptomatic without it and be switched from nasal to mouthpiece interfaces for daytime NVS as needed.
- Volume rather than pressure preset ventilation is used for patients who can air stack.
- Bilevel PAP used at high (ventilatory support) spans is reserved only for patients who cannot afford portable ventilators.
- Because many CNVS-dependent patients with SMA type 1 have no bulbar-innervated muscle function, clearly tracheostomy tubes are unnecessary for respiratory support even in the total absence of bulbar-innervated muscle function unless central nervous system/upper motor neuron hypertonicity results in inadequate upper airway patency for MIE to clear airway secretions as necessary.
- Of all the neuromuscular diseases, insufficient upper airway patency for effective mechanical in-exsufflation and, therefore, eventual need for tracheotomy only occurs for patients with ALS.
- At least for patients with DMD for which a large historically controlled study is available, patients live 10 years longer using CNVS than TMV.

*Sir Patrick: Don't misunderstand me, my boy, I'm not belittling your discovery. Most discoveries are made regularly every 15 years; and it's fully a hundred and fifty since yours was made last. That's something to be proud of…*

*—George Bernard Shaw in "The Doctor's Dilemma" 1906, a novel about the moral dilemmas created by limited resources and the conflicts between the demands of private medicine as a business and as a vocation. Things have not changed very much.*

The author has no commercial or financial conflicts of interest to report.
This work was not supported by any external funding.
[a] Department of Physical Medicine and Rehabilitation, Rutgers University New Jersey Medical School, Behavioral Health Building, F5759, 60 Orange Avenue, Newark, NJ 07103, USA; [b] Center for Mechanical Ventilation Alternatives and Pulmonary Rehabilitation, University Hospital, 150 Bergen Street, Newark, NJ 07103, USA
* Center for Mechanical Ventilation Alternatives and Pulmonary Rehabilitation, University Hospital, 150 Bergen Street, Newark, NJ 07103.
E-mail address: bachjr@njms.rutgers.edu

## HISTORICAL PERSPECTIVE
### Polysomnography and Sleep-Disordered Breathing

Although it was known for 50 years that the brain emitted electrical signals, it was not until 1929 that the German psychiatrist Hans Berger demonstrated electroencephalographic differences between sleep and wakefulness for humans.[1] In 1956 Bickelmann and colleagues[2] defined the pickwickian syndrome. Then in the early 1960s polysomnography including $CO_2$ measurements was performed for patients with the classic symptoms of sleep-disordered breathing (SDB).[3] In 1965 Gastaut and colleagues[4] reported that obstructive and mixed obstructive/central events rather than hypercapnia were the causes of hypersomnolence and other symptoms. As a result, $CO_2$ measurements were discontinued in favor of simple nasal airflow. Publications in 1969 and 1970 reported relief of symptoms by tracheostomy, further supporting the idea that airway obstruction was the problem.[5,6] In 1972 Christian Guilleminault introduced the monitoring of cardiorespiratory parameters[7]; and in 1974 Jerome Holland coined the term "polysomnogram."[8] Therefore, despite Charles Dickens' classic description of SDB in his novel David Copperfield in 1850, SDB was essentially "discovered" more than 100 years later.

In 1876 von Hauke[9] of Austria applied continuous negative airway pressure and continuous positive airway pressure (CPAP) using a chest shell. He also administered CPAP via an oronasal interface to treat atelectasis.[10] His work was forgotten until the late 1930s when Poulton and Barach independently used CPAP for treating acute pulmonary edema. Then in 1974 CPAP was delivered to 20 newborns with respiratory distress syndrome.[11] In 1981 Sullivan and coworkers[12] published CPAP outcomes for five patients with SDB. Once CPAP interfaces (masks) became commercially available in 1984, along with polysomnography to diagnosis and guide in its treatment, the CPAP treatment paradigm for SDB became widely accepted.

Besides increasing functional residual capacity, CPAP acts as a pneumatic splint to keep the upper airway open so that patients can use their inspiratory muscles to ventilate their lungs. It does not, however, provide ventilatory assistance, that is, support for inadequate inspiratory muscle force such as occurs for those with obesity-hypoventilation syndrome, postpoliomyelitis survivors, spinal cord injury (SCI), critical care neuromyopathy, or neuromuscular disease (NMD). Indeed, the failure of CPAP at any pressure to aid obesity-hypoventilation patients who have both airflow obstruction and insufficient inspiratory muscle force for their increased work of breathing induced Respironics Inc (Murrysville, PA) to develop bilevel positive airway pressure (PAP) and place their "BiPAP-ST machine" on the market in 1990. By permitting the independent adjustment of inspiratory positive airway pressure (IPAP) and expiratory positive airway pressure (EPAP), their machines provide ventilatory assistance as a function of the IPAP EPAP span. Thus, they are used as pressure preset ventilators and can provide full ventilatory support if used at spans of at least 18 cm $H_2O$ or more, but because they had no security alarms or internal or external battery function they have not been sanctioned for use for ventilatory support.

### Noninvasive Ventilation Versus Noninvasive Ventilatory Support

The goal of sleep doctors has been to titrate away apneas and hypopneas using noninvasive ventilation (NIV), a term that has become synonymous with CPAP and bilevel PAP at the lowest effective bilevel PAP spans. This is typically the approach used for patients with NMD. As a result the polysomnograms performed on them do not typically include $CO_2$ monitoring and their symptoms are attributed to central and obstructive events because polysomnographies are programmed to interpret every apnea and hypopnea as being caused by central or obstructive events rather than inspiratory muscle dysfunction. Irrespective of how weak they are, patients with NMD are often prescribed or extubated to bilevel PAP scans less than 10 cm $H_2O$ or inadequate for full ventilatory support.

Because other than for my papers nowhere else in the medical literature do the benefits of NIV include noninvasive ventilatory support (NVS), it is now time to coin a new term and abbreviation. Indeed, I have had a patient with NMD referred to me unsuccessfully attempting to use 23 cm $H_2O$ IPAP and 19 cm $H_2O$ EPAP. It would have been less uncomfortable to breathe in a hurricane. After switching him and other similarly managed patients to volume preset or in his case pressure preset ventilation at 23 cm $H_2O$ with no EPAP or positive end-expiratory pressure (PEEP), their daytime and sleep $CO_2$ normalized, symptoms were alleviated, and with progressive disease they eventually became dependent on continuous NVS (CNVS) without ever developing acute respiratory failure (ARF), being hospitalized, or needing a tracheostomy tube.

## PARADIGM SHIFTS TO TRACHEOSTOMY MECHANICAL VENTILATION AND NONINVASIVE POSITIVE PRESSURE VENTILATORY SUPPORT

From 1948 to 1952, a total of 3500 patients with poliomyelitis were treated at Los Angeles General Hospital. Of these, 15% to 20% used iron lungs for ventilatory support. Fatality rates decreased by placing tracheostomy tubes for airway suctioning (not for ventilatory support) and by better nursing care, especially when the Cof-flator (OEM Company, Hartford, CT) became available around 1954 (**Fig. 1**).[13,14] Meanwhile, over a 6-month period in 1952 in Denmark 316 of 866 cases of paralytic polio required ventilatory support, 70 at any particular time, with only one iron lung and six chest shell ventilators to support them. Dr Lassen then had indwelling tracheostomy tubes placed and 200 medical and dental students squeezing rubber bags to ventilate via the tubes around-the-clock for 3 or 4 months until the Danish Pulsula positive pressure ventilator became available. Continuous tracheostomy mechanical ventilation (TMV) facilitated the mobilization of these patients by permitting them to leave iron lungs for wheelchairs behind which the Pulsula could be rolled. As a result tracheotomy also became the convention in the United States. However, in 1953 Dr Affeldt of Rancho Los Amigos Hospital in California wrote that patients can have a simple mouthpiece "hang in the mouth, we even had one patient who has no breathing ability who has fallen asleep and been adequately ventilated by this procedure...You just hang it by the patients and they grip it with their lips, when they want it, and when they don't want it, they let go of it" (**Fig. 2**).[15] Like Dr Affeldt in Rancho, Dr Augusta Alba at Goldwater Memorial Hospital in New York City discovered that mouthpiece NVS users would nap without losing the mouthpieces and suffering respiratory arrest and all of the Goldwater patients,

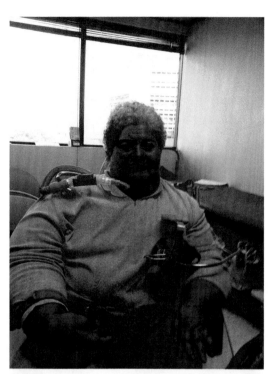

Fig. 2. Postpolio survivor dependent on CNVS, including daytime mouthpiece CNVS as seen here, for 62 years.

too, left body ventilators in favor of continuous mouthpiece CNVS.

The air for NVS was initially delivered via powerful blowers. The patient would take as much air as desired and let the rest blow mostly into their faces. When they slept their sleep was no doubt greatly disturbed because the blower was not a cycling ventilator and transient arousals were necessary to reflexively grab the mouthpiece for sleep NVS. However, although many patients had no autonomous breathing ability, no use of their limbs, no alarms on the blowers, and there was nothing holding the mouthpiece in the mouth other than their own oropharyngeal muscles and these muscles are not thought to function during random eye movement sleep, no deaths were reported.

In 1956 the Thompson Company (Boulder, CO) manufactured the 28-lb Bantam portable ventilator in a small suitcase (**Fig. 3**). The first Bantams were pressure control only and had no alarms or internal batteries but hundreds of patients used them indefinitely, in some cases for CNVS for up to 52 years. Many of these patients had 0 mL of vital capacity (VC) and no autonomous ability to breathe other than in some cases by glossopharyngeal breathing.[16–19] In 1960 mouthpiece NVS was cited in a review of mechanical ventilation.[20]

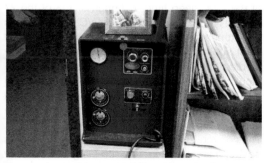

**Fig. 1.** Circa 1953 OEM Cof-flator (Hartford, Connecticut) from the author's collection.

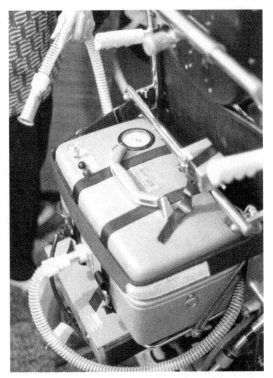

**Fig. 3.** Bantam pressure control ventilator (Thompson Company).

Then, in 1964 after the Bennett mouthpiece with Lipseal retention (Mallincrodt, Pleasanton, CA) became available for pulmonary function testing (**Fig. 4**),[21] Dr Alba convinced most of her nocturnal mouthpiece NVS users to use the Lipseal to secure the mouthpiece during sleep. The Lipseal prevented the mouthpiece from falling out of the mouth and its phalange sealed the lips, thereby reducing oral air leakage and oxyhemoglobin desaturations during sleep.[21]

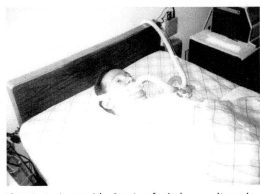

**Fig. 4.** Patient with 0 mL of vital capacity using mouthpiece with Lipseal retention for sleep and CNVS for 52 years.

None of the hundreds of CNVS-dependent patients in more than 20 centers around the world who rely on CNVS instead of tracheostomy tubes for continuous ventilatory support receive EPAP or PEEP and, clearly, none of them need it.[22] Indeed, EPAP/PEEP cannot be maintained during waking hours with patients using open systems of NVS and use during sleep results in leak compensation that tends to unnecessarily disturb sleep and can cause ventilators to auto-cycle. The EPAP or PEEP is also uncomfortable, hinders exhalation, unnecessarily increases intrathoracic pressure and decreases venous return, and necessitates higher inspiratory pressures for ventilatory assistance/support.

## MECHANISMS OF ACTION
### Conventional Approaches

Investigators typically list the many benefits of NIV, typically low spans of bilevel PAP or CPAP, yet admit to not understanding how it works. For example, "competing theories includ(e) resting of chronically fatigued respiratory muscles, increasing the compliance of the respiratory system by increased tidal volumes, reducing the load against which the respiratory muscle pump must work, resetting of respiratory centers at a more physiologic value of $Paco_2$, improving quality of sleep and avoiding cardiovascular consequences of repeated or prolonged nocturnal desaturations."[23] Everything is often considered except that, at least for patients with 0 mL of VC, the open systems of NIV can be used for NVS just as can TMV.

### Noninvasive Approaches

For open systems to provide NVS, full ventilatory support settings need to be used and CNS reflex activity during sleep sufficiently effective to eliminate excessive leak.[24,25] In a study of CNVS-dependent patients using nocturnal mouthpiece NVS, expiratory passage of air through the nose occurred during an average of only 33% ± 27% of the total sleep time. Although only 3 of the 27 Lipseal NVS users had sufficient VC for 10 minutes of autonomous breathing ability when supine, all slept supine, 22 (82%) of the nocturnal oximetry studies yielded normal (>95%) mean oxyhemoglobin saturation ($Spo_2$), and 12 of 15 had maximum end-tidal $CO_2$ ($EtCO_2$) levels less than 45 mm Hg. Previous sawtooth patterns of severe desaturations smoothed out and normalized. Thus, mouthpiece/Lipseal NVS normalizes nocturnal ventilation by creating a partially closed system to ventilate the lungs. For 13 nocturnal mouthpiece/Lipseal NVS users undergoing inpatient polysomnography, the time periods in the deeper sleep stages tended to be normal as a percentage of sleep period time.[26] Of the five who had a mean $Spo_2$ less than 95% for 1 hour or more of sleep, three of the five used mouthpiece NVS without a Lipseal or with inadequate Lipseal retention.[26]

In 1987 we reported the use of CNVS for a patient with no autonomous ability to breathe and 100 mL of VC,[27] and in 1990 reported normalization of sleep alveolar ventilation and daytime blood gases for 34 patients with NMDs by nocturnal nasal NVS including 16 who were CNVS dependent.[28] Since 1989 our sleep $EtCO_2$ and oximetry studies have continued to demonstrate adequate alveolar ventilation to alleviate hypoventilation symptoms whether using Lipseal or nasal NVS.[24,28]

Open systems of NVS delivered during sleep via simple mouthpiece or nasal interfaces are less effective or ineffective for patients receiving supplemental $O_2$, heavy sedation, or narcotics.[19,29] In 1995 we demonstrated that oral leakage of patients using nasal NVS during sleep is increased when nasal NVS users are placed on supplemental $O_2$ or sedative medications.[30] Indeed, for patients with severe cardiopulmonary diseases who do require high levels of supplemental $O_2$ it is generally reported that nasal NIV does not generally succeed in averting intubation more than 70% of the time.[31] We speculate that this is explained in large part by failure of central nervous system–mediated activity to decrease insufflation leakage when normal $Spo_2$ is artificially maintained. Therefore, for patients with severe pulmonary restrictive disorders caused by inspiratory muscle weakness or paralysis but who have normal lung physiology, excessive insufflation leakage that could cause recurrence of symptoms and hypoventilation is prevented by the brain remaining alert during sleep to prevent excessive prolonged leakage.[25]

## The Two Paradigms

### Conventional noninvasive ventilation to tracheostomy

In the conventional NIV to tracheotomy paradigm, patients with progressive inspiratory muscle dysfunction are referred for polysomnograms to evaluate for SDB and treated with CPAP or low-span bilevel PAP with the least expensive CPAP interfaces and often without giving the patient a choice of interfaces. Some have recommended initiation of bilevel PAP with $Pco_2$ of 45 mm Hg.[32] Because $Pco_2$ increases about 4 mm Hg during sleep, $Pco_2$ of 49 to 55 mm Hg has also been proposed as threshold to indicate introduction of sleep bilevel PAP for the NMD

population.[33,34] Because asymptomatic normal patients can at times have $Paco_2$ elevations to 55 mm Hg during sleep, the American Academy of Sleep Medicine suggests that $CO_2$ levels exceed 55 mm Hg for at least 10 minutes during sleep to justify a diagnosis of sleep hypoventilation.[35] Indeed, we have found that many patients become symptomatic with sleep $CO_2$ somewhat lower than this but measurement of $Pco_2$ during sleep, along with spirometry, $Spo_2$ monitoring, and especially symptomatology should all be taken into account when considering initiation of sleep ventilation and to justify the decision to third-party payers.[36,37] Supplemental $O_2$ should be avoided for these patients.

VC less than 50% of predicted normal is another conventional indication to introduce bilevel PAP. However, using pulmonary function as guidelines to indicate need for NIV is suboptimal because we have had patients with amyotrophic lateral sclerosis (ALS) with 90% of predicted normal VC, when sitting, who were CNVS dependent, whereas others with VC of 300 mL or about 5% of normal are symptom-free without any ventilator use.

Once bilevel PAP is introduced, apnea and hypopnea titrations are often repeated as patients weaken with advancing disease or age. If patients become symptomatic because the bilevel PAP becomes inadequate or if they become dyspneic when attempting to discontinue NIV or extend NIV into daytime hours they are informed that they need tracheostomy tubes. Many develop ARF during intercurrent chest colds and require intubation once $CO_2$ levels skyrocket following $O_2$ administration.[17] When unable to pass spontaneous breathing trials or pass ventilator weaning parameters they are told that they need tracheostomy tubes rather than be extubated to CNVS and mechanical insufflation-exsufflation (MIE) to expulse airway secretions.[38,39]

### Noninvasive ventilatory support

Once respiratory muscle dysfunction is documented by diminished supine VC, hypercapnia, and so forth, and there are symptoms from respiratory muscle dysfunction and/or hypoventilation,[28] sleep nasal NVS is introduced. We and others[22] believe that only symptoms should indicate sleep NVS for adolescents and adults and mainly paradoxic breathing indicate it for infants. When symptoms are questionable sleep $Spo_2$ and $CO_2$ studies are undertaken and abnormal results are used to convince patients to try sleep nasal NVS and third-party payers to pay for it. When dyspnea occurs when attempting to discontinue nasal NVS in the morning, we encourage patients to extend NVS into daytime hours as necessary but introduce them to mouthpiece NVS for waking hours. For intercurrent episodes of ARF requiring intubation, irrespective of extent of respiratory muscle dysfunction, they are routinely extubated to CNVS and MIE and return home using CNVS rather than undergoing tracheotomy.[28,40]

From what we learned from the many hundreds of iron lung/body ventilator users switched to NVS,[25] from more than 1000 CNVS-dependent patients in our center,[40] and from the more than 700 with Duchenne muscular dystrophy (DMD), ALS, and spinal muscular atrophy (SMA) type 1 being managed by CNVS in centers around the world,[22] patients symptomatic for SDB but whose symptoms are caused by inspiratory muscle weakness rather than central or obstructive events can be placed on volume-preset NVS that is generally provided via active ventilator circuits from portable volume-preset ventilators for sleep or daytime NVS. Full ventilatory support settings are used to optimally rest inspiratory muscles during sleep, to normalize daytime and sleep $CO_2$, and to relieve symptoms without need for apnea and hypopnea titrations or any polysomnographies at all. Indeed, apnea-hypopnea indices can be minimal or high irrespective of $CO_2$ levels.

We have typically prescribed delivered volumes of 800 to 1500 mL for adolescents and adults for 40 years for NVS and let the user choose the desired volumes to physiologically varying tidal volumes.[40] We prefer pressure-preset ventilation at about 18 cm $H_2O$ for small children and others who cannot air stack for active lung volume recruitment (LVR).[41] Because the indication for initiating sleep nasal NVS is relief of symptoms, full batteries of pulmonary function testing are unnecessary. Pulmonary function testing typically excludes active and passive LVR,[42] cough flows,[43] $CO_2$ measurements, and supine VC. The latter is most important because it is during sleep that hypercapnia generally begins and normalizing sleep ventilation relieves symptoms.

Likewise, polysomnograms are unnecessary because they do not access for respiratory muscle weakness and bilevel PAP titrations are unnecessary. Sleep $Spo_2$ and $EtCO_2$ or transcutaneous $CO_2$ monitoring can be done and if clearly abnormal,[44] especially with $CO_2$ levels reaching 50 mm Hg or more, the patient is encouraged to try nasal NVS for sleep. If they derive no perceived benefit from it or if the benefit is insufficient to justify the inconvenience of using it, they are informed to return for re-evaluation generally in 3 months for patients with ALS or in 12 months for others.

Small pediatric patients often have normal or apnea-hypopnea indices less than two yet can present with severe paradoxic breathing and flushing, perspiration, and poor-quality sleep. All infants with NMDs who have paradoxic breathing need to be placed on sleep nasal NVS to reverse paradoxicing[45] and to relieve the flushing and perspiration. Nocturnal nasal NVS for these small children promotes normal lung and chest wall compliance and growth,[46] and prevents pectus excavatum and other chest wall deformities.[45]

## ANCILLARY TECHNIQUES TO OPTIMIZE LUNG HEALTH AND LONG-TERM NONINVASIVE VENTILATORY SUPPORT
### Lung Volume Recruitment

LVR is essential to maintain or increase pulmonary compliance and lung volumes, and to increase cough flows and improve speech volume.[47,48] The LVR is administered passively or actively. Daily routine passive LVR is delivered via a mouthpiece, nasal, or oronasal interface. Mouthpiece LVR was probably first performed in the 1950s when CNVS users turned up the pressures on their Bantams to get deep lung volumes to shout, cough, and mobilize lung tissues. In 1969 Dr Augusta Alba described the maximum passive LVR attained this way as the "artificial inspiratory capacity."[21] We now refer to this as the "lung insufflation capacity."[48]

Active LVR or air stacking may have first been described in 1966 when Kirby and coworkers[49] reported that cough peak flows could be doubled and readily exceed 6 L/s for many SCI patients by receiving and holding consecutively delivered volumes of air to the maximum volume that could be held by the glottis (air stacking).

### Manually and Mechanically Assisted Coughing

Assisted cough peak flows are achieved from the deep lung volumes created by air stacking by applying an abdominal or thoracoabdominal thrust concomitantly with glottis opening.[49] The increase in cough peak flows achieved by manually assisted coughing to expulse airway debris and maintain or return $Spo_2$ to normal (>94%) can make the difference between an otherwise benign upper respiratory tract infection developing into pneumonia and ARF that necessitates hospitalization, intubation, and conventional recourse to tracheotomy or the patient simply being treated effectively at home using NVS, manually assisted coughing, and possibly MIE to maintain normal $Spo_2$.[50]

Mechanically assisted coughing is simply the use of MIE at pressures of 50 to 60 cm $H_2O$ via the mouth or mouth and nose (oronasal interface) or at 60 to 70 cm $H_2O$ via any invasive airway tubes. For babies the same pressures are used but because they breathe so quickly the insufflation and exsufflation must either be timed to the child's breathing or the Cough-Trak of the T70 CoughAssist (Philips-Respironics, Inc, Murrysville, PA) used for the child to trigger the machine.[22]

## COMPARISON OF NONINVASIVE VENTILATION/INVASIVE VERSUS NONINVASIVE MANAGEMENT PARADIGMS

No patients want invasive airway tubes and NVS is preferred over TMV for swallowing, speech, comfort, appearance, security, and overall by patients who have used both.[51] Cognitively intact respirator-dependent patients with healthy lungs whose $SpO_2$ baseline is greater than 94% in ambient air despite respiratory muscle weakness or paralysis do not need tracheostomy tubes if managed by CNVS and proper use of MIE (Cough-Assist) to clear airway secretions when necessary.[36] Despite numerous controlled studies in the neurology literature that report minimal prolongations of "tracheostomy-free" survival by using sleep NIV versus no NIV, the reported prolongations are insignificant by comparison with tracheostomy-free survival by CNVS dependence for 30 years to age 53 (mean, 40 years) for DMD patients,[52,53] more than 20 years of CNVS dependence for patients with SMA type 1 who have been CNVS dependent since 4 months of age with 0 mL of VC and only residual autonomous movements of the eyes (**Figs. 5** and **6**),[41,54] for decades of CNVS dependence for patients with milder SMAs,[55] more than 60 years of CNVS dependence for postpoliomyelitis survivors (see **Fig. 2**),[35] and 40 years for high-level SCI patients.[21,40]

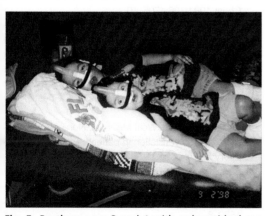

**Fig. 5.** Brothers ages 3 and 1 with only residual eye movements and no autonomous breathing ability CNVS dependent since 8 and 4 months of age, respectively.

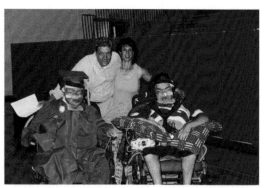

**Fig. 6.** The same brothers now aged 20 and 18 years with 0 mL of vital capacity and CNVS dependent since infancy. Note that they have successfully used nasal CNVS despite having all nutrition via nasogastric tubes since 4 months of age.

In summary, patients with weak or paralyzed respiratory muscles should only be prescribed and use sleep nasal NVS when symptomatic without it and be switched from nasal to mouthpiece interfaces for daytime NVS as needed. Pressure-preset ventilation can be used for patients who cannot air stack but bilevel PAP use at high spans reserved only for patients who cannot afford portable ventilators. Because many of our CNVS-dependent patients with SMA type 1 have no bulbar-innervated muscle function, clearly tracheostomy tubes are unnecessary for respiratory support even in the total absence of bulbar-innervated muscle function unless central nervous system/upper motor neuron hypertonicity results in inadequate upper airway patency for MIE to clear airway secretions as necessary. This only occurs for patients with ALS but in no other NMD.[21] Although it may be surprising to some that patients consider CNVS to be safer than TMV, it should be appreciated that 70% of CNVS users with intact bulbar-innervated musculature can master glossopharyngeal breathing sufficiently to breathe without ventilator use despite having little or no VC.[56] This security is impossible for patients with TMV who necessarily fear accidental disconnections and ventilator failure. Also, at least for patients with DMD for which a large historically controlled study is available, patients live 10 years longer using CNVS than TMV.[57]

## REFERENCES

1. Berger H. Uber das elektroenenkeephalogramm des menschen on the human electroencephalogram. Arch Psychiatr Nervenkr 1929;87:527–70 [in German].

2. Bickelmann AG, Burwell CS, Robin ED, et al. Extreme obesity associated with alveolar hypoventilation; a pickwickian syndrome. Am J Med 1956; 21(5):811–8.

3. Deak M, Epstein LJ. The history of polysomnography. Sleep Med Clin 2009;4:313–21.

4. Gastaut H, Tassinari CA, Duron B. Polygraphic study of diurnal and nocturnal (hypnic and respiratory) episodal manifestations of Pickwick syndrome. Rev Neurol (Paris) 1965;112(6):568–79 [in French].

5. Kuhlo W, Doll E, Franck MC. Successful management of pickwickian syndrome using long-term tracheostomy. Dtsch Med Wochenschr 1969;94(24): 1286–90 [in German].

6. Lugaresi E, Coccagna G, Mantovani M, et al. Effects of tracheotomy in hypersomnia with periodic respiration. Rev Neurol (Paris) 1970;123(4):267–8 [in French].

7. Dement WC. History of sleep physiology and medicine. In: Kryger MH, Roth T, Dement W, editors. Principles and practice of sleep medicine. 4th edition. Philadelphia: Elsevier; 2005. p. 1–12.

8. Atkinson JW. The evolution of polysomnographic technology. In: Butkov N, Lee-Chiong T, editors. Fundamentals of sleep technology. Philadelphia: Lippincott, Williams & Wilkins; 2007. p. 1–9.

9. Von Hauke I. Der pneumatische panzer. Beitrag zur mechanischen behandlung der brustkrankheiten, vol. 15. Vienna, Austria: Wiener Medizinische Presse; 1874. p. 785–836.

10. Waldenburg L. Die pneumatische behandlung der respirations und circulationskrankheiten im anschluss an die pneumatometrie und spirometrie. Hirschwald, Berlin, 1880, p 420 cited in Woollam CHM. The development of apparatus for intermittent negative pressure respiration: 1832-1918. Anaesthesia 1976;31:537–47.

11. Dunn PM, Thearle MJ, Parsons AC, et al. Use of the 'Gregory box' (CPAP) in treatment of RDS of the newborn: preliminary report. Arch Dis Child 1972; 47:674–5.

12. Sullivan CE, Issa FG, Berthon-Jones M, et al. Reversal of obstructive sleep apnoea by continuous positive airway pressure applied through the nares. Lancet 1981;8225(1):862–5.

13. Hodes HL. Treatment of respiratory difficulty in poliomyelitis. In: Poliomyelitis: papers and discussions presented at the third international poliomyelitis conference. Philadelphia: Lippincott; 1955. p. 91–113.

14. Barach AL, Beck GJ, Smith WH. Mechanical production of expiratory flow rates surpassing the capacity of human coughing. Am J Med Sci 1953; 226:241–8.

15. Round Table Conference on Poliomyelitis Equipment, Roosevelt Hotel, New York City, May 28-29, 1953, National Foundation for Infantile Paralysis-March of Dimes, Inc., White Plains, NY.

16. Dail CW, Affeldt JE. Glossopharyngeal breathing [video]. Los Angeles (CA): Department of Visual Education, College of Medical Evangelists; 1954.

17. Bach JR, Alba AS, Bodofsky E, et al. Glossopharyngeal breathing and non-invasive aids in the management of post-polio respiratory insufficiency. Birth Defects 1987;23(4):99–113.

18. Dail CW. Glossopharyngeal breathing by paralyzed patients. Calif Med 1951;75:217.

19. Bach JR, Alba AS, Saporito LR. Intermittent positive pressure ventilation via the mouth as an alternative to tracheostomy for 257 ventilator users. Chest 1993;103(1):174–82.

20. Allen WC. Therapists must become more expert as use of respiratory aids. Inhal Ther 1960;5(1):20–8.

21. Alba A, Solomon M, Trainor FS. Management of respiratory insufficiency in spinal cord lesions, In: Proceedings of the 17th Veteran's Administration Spinal Cord Injury Conference, July 7, 1969, Las Vegas, NV. p. 200–213.

22. Gonçalves MR, Bach JR, Ishikawa Y, et al. Continuous noninvasive ventilatory support outcomes for neuromuscular disease: a multicenter collaboration and literature review. Rev Port Pneumol. In press.

23. Gonzalez-Bermejo J, Perrin C, Janssens JP, et al. Proposal for a systemic analysis of polygraphy or polysomnography for identifying and scoring abnormal events occurring during non-invasive ventilation. Thorax 2012;67:546–52.

24. Bach JR, Alba AS, Shin D. Management alternatives for post-polio respiratory insufficiency: assisted ventilation by nasal or oral-nasal interface. Am J Phys Med Rehabil 1989;68(12):264–71.

25. Bach JR, Penek J. Obstructive sleep apnea complicating negative pressure ventilatory support in patients with chronic paralytic/restrictive ventilatory dysfunction. Chest 1991;99(6):1386–93.

26. Bach JR, Alba AS. Sleep and nocturnal mouthpiece IPPV efficiency in post poliomyelitis ventilator users. Chest 1994;106:1705–10.

27. Bach JR, Alba AS, Mosher R, et al. Intermittent positive pressure ventilation via nasal access in the management of respiratory insufficiency. Chest 1987;92(7):168–70.

28. Bach JR, Alba AS. Management of chronic alveolar hypoventilation by nasal ventilation. Chest 1990; 97(1):52–7.

29. Wysocki M, Tric L, Wolff MA, et al. Noninvasive pressure support ventilation in patients with acute respiratory failure. Chest 1993;103:907–13.

30. Bach JR, Robert D, Leger P, et al. Sleep fragmentation in kyphoscoliotic individuals with alveolar hypoventilation treated by nasal IPPV. Chest 1995;107(6): 1552–8.

31. McNeill GBS, Glossop AJ. Clinical applications of non-invasive ventilation in critical care. Br J Anesth Education 2012;12(1):33–7.

32. Ozsancak A, D'Ambrosio C, Hill NS. Nocturnal noninvasive ventilation. Chest 2008;133:1275–86.

33. Ward S, Chatwin M, Heather S, et al. Randomised controlled trial of non-invasive ventilation (NIV) for nocturnal hypoventilation in neuromuscular and chest wall disease patients with daytime normocapnia. Thorax 2005;60:1019–24.

34. Berry RB, Budhiraja R, Gottlieb DJ, et al. Rules for scoring respiratory events in sleep: update of the 2007 AASM manual for the scoring of sleep and associated events: deliberations of the sleep apnea definitions task force of the American Academy of Sleep Medicine. J Clin Sleep Med 2012; 8(5):597–619.

35. Bach JR, Mehta AD. Respiratory muscle aids to avert respiratory failure and tracheostomy: a new patient management paradigm. J Neurorestoratalogy 2014; 2:25–35.

36. Kang SW. Pulmonary rehabilitation in patients with neuromuscular disease. Yonsei Med J 2006;47: 307–14.

37. Chiou M, Bach JR, Saporito LR, et al. Quantitation of oxygen induced hypercapnia in respiratory pump failure. Rev Port Pneumol (2006) 2016;22(5):262–5.

38. Bach JR, Sinquee D, Saporito LR, et al. Efficacy of mechanical insufflation-exsufflation in extubating unweanable subjects with restrictive pulmonary disorders. Respir Care 2015;60(4):477–83.

39. Bach JR, Gonçalves MR, Hamdani I, et al. Extubation of unweanable patients with neuromuscular weakness: a new management paradigm. Chest 2010;137(5):1033–9.

40. Bach JR. The management of patients with neuromuscular disease. Philadelphia: Elsevier; 2004. p. 414.

41. Bach JR, Gupta K, Reyna M, et al. Spinal muscular atrophy type 1: prolongation of survival by noninvasive respiratory aids. Pediatric Asthma Allergy Immunol 2009;22(4):151–62.

42. Chiou M, Bach JR, Jethani L, et al. Lung volume recruitment and vital capacity in Duchenne muscular dystrophy. J Rehabil Med 2017;49(1): 49–53.

43. Kang SW, Bach JR. Maximum insufflation capacity: vital capacity and cough flows in neuromuscular disease. Am J Phys Med Rehabil 2000;79(3):222–7.

44. Won YH, Choi WA, Lee JW, et al. Sleep transcutaneous vs. end-tidal $CO2$ monitoring for patients with neuromuscular disease. Am J Phys Med Rehabil 2016;95(2):91–5.

45. Bach JR, Bianchi C. Prevention of pectus excavatum for children with spinal muscular atrophy type 1. Am J Phys Med Rehabil 2003;82(10):815–9.

46. Bach JR, Kang SW. Disorders of ventilation: weakness, stiffness, and mobilization. Chest 2000; 117(2):301–3.

47. Kang SW, Bach JR. Maximum insufflation capacity. Chest 2000;118(1):61–5.

48. Bach JR, Mahajan K, Lipa B, et al. Lung insufflation capacity in neuromuscular disease. Am J Phys Med Rehabil 2008;87(9):720–5.

49. Kirby NA, Barnerias MJ, Siebens AA. An evaluation of assisted cough in quadriparetic patients. Arch Phys Med Rehabil 1966;47:705–10.

50. Bach JR, Martinez D. Duchenne muscular dystrophy: prolongation of survival by noninvasive interventions. Respir Care 2011;56(6):744–50.

51. Bach JR. A comparison of long-term ventilatory support alternatives from the perspective of the patient and care giver. Chest 1993;104(6):1702–6.

52. Bach JR, Tran J, Durante S. Cost and physician effort analysis of invasive vs. noninvasive respiratory management of Duchenne muscular dystrophy. Am J Phys Med Rehabil 2015;94(6):474–82.

53. Villanova M, Kazibwe S. New survival target for Duchenne muscular dystrophy. Am J Phys Med Rehabil 2017;96(2):e28–30.

54. Bach JR, Bakshiyev R, Hon A. Noninvasive respiratory management for patients with spinal cord injury and neuromuscular disease. Tanaffos J 2012;11(1): 7–11.

55. Bach JR, Tuccio MC, Khan U, et al. Vital capacity in spinal muscular atrophy. Am J Phys Med Rehabil 2012;91(6):487–93.

56. Bach JR, Alba AS. Noninvasive options for ventilatory support of the traumatic high level quadriplegic. Chest 1990;98(3):613–9.

57. Ishikawa Y, Miura T, Ishikawa Y, et al. Duchenne muscular dystrophy: survival by cardio-respiratory interventions. Neuromuscul Disord 2011;21:47–51.

# Future of Positive Airway Pressure Technology

Karin G. Johnson, MD[a],*, David M. Rapoport, MD[b]

## KEYWORDS

• Positive airway pressure • Obstructive sleep apnea • Central sleep apnea • Noninvasive ventilation

## KEY POINTS

- Further technological improvements in positive airway pressure (PAP) technology will allow for smaller and more energy-efficient machines to improve tolerance and battery-powered options for travel and for countries without reliable power.
- Personalized PAP through machine learning and adjustable algorithms may improve treatment and tolerance to PAP.
- Incorporating data from other medical devices, such as insulin pumps and pacemakers, and with embedded or external sensors, such as ECG and oximetry, could increase understanding about the effects of PAP and which patients will benefit most and drive algorithms to improve treatment.
- Cross-platform integration of PAP data into electronic health record may enhance PAP utilization and optimization, provider documentation and research opportunities.
- The largest limitation of PAP technology may be not understanding the psychosocial issues that have so far prevented many patients from using it for the full 7 hours to 8 hours they need to sleep free of obstructive sleep apnea.

## INTRODUCTION

Continuous positive airway pressure (CPAP) has been around for 37 years. When first proposed, many suspected that its use in the clinical arena would be a transient phenomenon, because few people believed patients would be ready to accept a nasal mask for nightly use. To date, however, no therapy has come close to PAP's physiologic success for treating obstructive sleep apnea (OSA). Thus, it is widely used as a benchmark of physiologic research that requires reversal of upper airway obstruction in sleep; clinically, PAP remains the most widely recommended therapy for OSA.

Despite many technological advances in mask therapy, blower algorithms, and accessories like humidifiers, however, it is increasingly recognized that a major limitation of CPAP has been suboptimal adherence by a substantial minority of patients. This, rather than enhancing the effect on OSA physiology, has become the major focus for investigation and it is likely that the future of PAP technology will depend on addressing (or accepting) this limitation. Several areas of investigation are actively being pursued and others are being discussed.

This article discusses the future of PAP technology. The focus is on (1) technology improvements in the delivery of PAP; (2) improvements in PAP

Financial Disclosures: Dr K.G. Johnson has no relevant financial conflicts of interest. She serves on the policy committee of the American Academy of Sleep Medicine. Dr D.M. Rapoport receives royalties for intellectual property relating to CPAP and research support from Fisher and Paykel Healthcare, grant support from the NIH/CDC and sits on advisory boards for BioMarin and Cortex Pharmaceuticals.

[a] Department of Neurology, University of Massachusetts Medical School-Baystate, Baystate Medical Center, Neurodiagnostics and Sleep Center, 759 Chestnut Street, Wesson Ground, Springfield, MA 01199, USA; [b] Division of Pulmonary, Critical Care and Sleep Medicine, Icahn School of Medicine at Mt. Sinai, One Gustave L. Levy Place, Annenberg Building, Room A5-20W, New York, NY 10029-6574, USA
* Corresponding author.
E-mail address: karin.johnson@bhs.org

Sleep Med Clin 12 (2017) 617–622
http://dx.doi.org/10.1016/j.jsmc.2017.08.001
1556-407X/17/© 2017 Elsevier Inc. All rights reserved.

algorithms; and (3) improvements in PAP informatics. Current limitations of PAP technology and whether technological improvements are sufficient to improve PAP beyond where it is today are discussed.

## TECHNOLOGY IMPROVEMENTS IN THE DELIVERY OF POSITIVE AIRWAY PRESSURE
### Blower Technology

Currently most PAP systems use direct current (DC) brushless motor blower technology, which limits the size and energy efficiency of current machines. **Fig. 1** shows several blower options studied for use in PAP technology.

Multistage DC brushless motors have multiple impellers to allow for higher flow at lower motor speeds, allowing for quieter motors that can achieve desired speeds more rapidly.[1]

Three-phase torque motors, such as the switch reluctance motor, work by cycling through 3 phases—1 negative current, 1 positive current, and 1 nonenergized—creating rotational torque.[2] Similar effects can be achieved with 3-phase electric motors using high-efficiency permanent magnets.[3]

A Roots-type blower is a multilobed positive displacement pump that works by trapping air in pockets to move it forward.[4] A bias valve closes the exhalation valve at the start of inspiration and regulates the positive end-expiratory pressure during exhalation. Power consumption is minimized when the bias pressure is able to be low and constant allowing for smaller, more efficient, battery-powered devices.

Microelectromechanical system (MEMS) technology is currently used in several medical devices, including hearing aids and insulin pumps. This technology is being developed by Marsh[5]

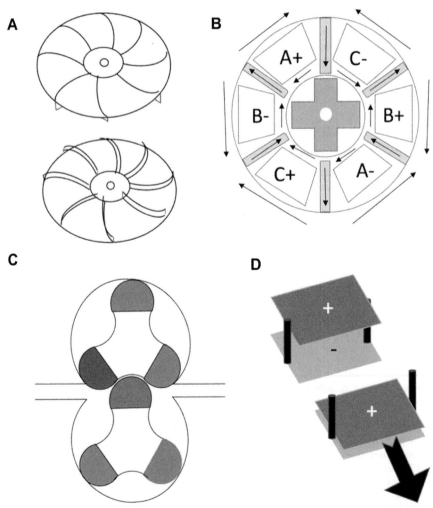

**Fig. 1.** Blower technology. (*A*) DC brushless multistage blower. (*B*) Three-stage torque motor. (*C*) Roots 3-lobed blower. (*D*) Electrostatic micro–air pump.

to create a disposable battery-powered CPAP that is a little bigger than a nasal pillow mask. Small air pumps are made with electrostatic membranes that move when voltage is applied, causing a bellows action to move air. Valves control the flow of air; the amount of voltage applied can alter the speed at which the pumps work. By placing many micropumps in parallel and activating the pumps thousands of times per second, adequate flow and pressure can be generated.[5] Unlike fan-style pumps, air pressure can be quickly turned on and off for quicker reactivity to flow changes.

MEMS technology can be applied with sensor and microprocessor technology so that functionalities, including ramp feature, expiratory pressure relief, autoCPAP, and bilevel PAP, are all possibilities.

## Humidifier Technology

Humidifiers are an important comfort element needed to increase PAP tolerance but limit the miniaturization of current machines. Waterless heat and moisture exchangers (HME) have been used for over 20 years in ventilated patients[6] and are now incorporated into the tubing (eg, AirMini [ResMed, San Diego, CA]). Heat and moisture exchangers wick moisture from exhaled air and then return the moisture to the air on inhalation. The same concept can be used by small humidifier chambers in which a small volume of water is placed in a chamber with a hydrophilic wick. By heating an element at one end of the wick, the amount of water that is vaporized as air is blown over it can be modulated.[7]

Systems without tubing can function without a bias leak, including smaller motors like MEMS air pumps that do not need 2 meter of tubing and can be mounted on the face. This approach decreases the flow through the system because it is not necessary to clear tubing dead space, thus greatly reducing the need for humidity in the system and also possibly decreasing dryness issues.

Autoadjustable humidity could adjust in response to leak when patient's are at higher risk for dryness. The machine could also query the patient in the AM about mouth dryness and subsequently adjust the following night's humidification level.

## Mask Technology

Mask technology has been a major focus of companies desiring to improve PAP adherence. Newer materials and designs, including memory foam, are used to improve seal. Customized masks

using 3-D printing are being developed. Smart masks that can sense when there is leak and move air pressure around to help seal the leak are another possibility. Masks could also be developed with microsensors using MEMS technology to track body position, pulse, transcutaneous $CO_2$ or end-tidal $CO_2$, or oxygen levels that can feedback to the PAP device and aid in diagnosis and home monitoring.

## Battery Technology

Currently PAP use is primarily limited to areas with reliable electricity. This can affect travel but more importantly is a significant limitation in large parts of the developing world where electricity is erratic or nonexistent. Battery advances, including metal-air batteries, such as zinc-air, aluminum-air, and lithium-air, have high-energy densities needed to provide long-lasting power in a small size. A built-in automatic transfer switch that allows PAP to switch from electrical power to a temporary battery if the utility source fails could also optimize battery use in places with some electricity.

## Cleaning Technology

The hassle of cleaning PAP equipment and the inability to clean the entire circuit are issues for many patients. Self-cleaning systems using UV light or a chemical cleaning system could be incorporated into the device.

## Feedback Modalities

Currently, almost all PAP systems are driven by sensed airflow in the blower, whether they are CPAP, bilevel PAP, adaptive servoventilation, or volume-assured pressure support. By using other sensors and data for feedback, algorithms can be enhanced.

**Box 1** lists future possible feedback signals and data that can be used to drive PAP algorithms if improved mask or machine sensor technology can be developed. ECG signal can be used not only as a marker of sympathetic activation but also for spectral analysis as a marker of sleep stability.[8,9] Devices could also allow for feedback from sensors worn during the day or long-term implanted sensors, such as with insulin pumps, pacemakers, or ventricular assist devices. Coordination with signals from implantable hypoglossal nerve stimulators may be used for patients who may require combination therapy.

Inertial motion capture, like Fitbit (San Francisco, CA), uses MEMS technology to miniaturize gyroscope and accelerometer functionality to determine position and movement data.

---

**Box 1**
**Future feedback data**

Oxygen saturations

End-tidal $CO_2$ or transcutaneous $CO_2$ levels

Lung function measures

    Lung resistance

    Lung elastance

    Airway compliance

    Peak expiratory flow

ECG

    Sleep stability

    Heart rate increases

Inertial motion capture

    Body position

    Actigraphy

Snore recordings

Physiologic sensors

    External sensors

    Insulin pumps

    Pacemakers and defibrillators

    Ventricular assist devices

Patient-reported outcomes

---

Forced oscillation technique currently used to differentiate central from obstructive apneas, combined with pressure, flow, and volume data, can also be used to determine information about a patient's lung function. PAP could report and incorporate lung resistance, elastance, compliance at both the central and conducting airways and the alveoli, forced expiratory volumes, forced expiratory flow, forced vital capacity and peak expiratory flow, and total and residual lung volumes into algorithms.[10]

## IMPROVEMENTS IN POSITIVE AIRWAY PRESSURE ALGORITHMS

Most current automatic titrating (auto) PAP systems adjust pressure to minimize surrogates of high airway resistance or airway collapse. These surrogate signals are often grouped under the concept of detecting the degree of flow limitation. It has been suggested that standardization of this parameter in both manual and automated analyses could result in improvement of the titration of CPAP, either initially or continuously. Other algorithms are being developed and studied as drivers for autotitration.[11,12]

### Machine Learning

Using samples from patients with particular clinical outcomes, artificial intelligence technology can be used to train the computer to find flow patterns that are most predictive of PAP (or other) therapy and these patterns may then influence autoCPAP technology.[13] An example of this is the ResMed algorithm that is purported to be specific to the flow patterns and nature of OSA specifically found in women.

PAP requirements vary from patient to patient and may differ in different stages of sleep and body positions and in response to other changes, such as nasal congestion. Algorithms exist and may continue to evolve that recognize these changes in patient state (eg, periods of wakefulness when CPAP is not needed or positional changes that may imply predictive changes in pressure). These algorithms may be merged further into the driver of pressure profiles. Although many patients can be treated with standard settings, other patients may benefit from customizable treatment beyond what current algorithms allow. Manual override of algorithms to set sensitivity levels for what the machine responds to and the speed of the response could also allow for further individualization, although it remains to be established that any "customization" of the PAP delivered will have an appreciable effect on overall usage.

Machine learning can be used to optimize settings throughout the night. Algorithms could learn what settings not only minimize events and improve oxygen or $CO_2$ levels but also which settings lead to the longest hours of use or the best patient-reported outcomes or other physiologic measures, as listed in **Box 1**. Body position sensors could allow the machine to learn what pressures are optimal in particular positions.

### Central Sleep Apnea Algorithms

Improved algorithms that adjust in response to periodic breathing and central apneas may further improve the treatment and tolerance in patients with complex sleep apnea. The Intellipap 2 AutoAdjust (DeVilbiss [Devilbiss Healthcare, Somerset, PA]) algorithm holds or reduces pressure in response to periodic breathing and central apneas. The Respironics (Murrysville, PA) autoCPAP algorithm has variable breathing and unresponsive apnea logic that also attempts to stabilize complex sleep apnea.[14]

Spectral analysis of pulse and respiratory rate data could also be used to distinguish between obstructive and central or complex physiology.[9] It may be learned that there are different physiologies, such as patients with short versus long event length or patients with tendencies toward mixed events who may better tolerate or benefit from different PAP adjustments.

## Automated and Adjustable Algorithms

Given there is a shortage of sleep medicine specialists, more patients are likely to be diagnosed and managed by primary care physicians. Automated algorithms to both optimize the treatment of more patients as well as alert the primary care physicians or other care provider when help from a specialist is needed will be critical to expanding care to the millions of untreated or undertreated patients.

Currently the algorithms for both autoCPAP and more advanced modalities are fixed by the vendor's algorithms. Future modalities could allow for more flexibility for a provider to control settings, such as sensitivity to flow characteristics or for adaptive machine learning to determine the optimal settings based on residual events and patient feedback.

## IMPROVEMENTS IN POSITIVE AIRWAY PRESSURE INFORMATICS
### Compliance Data Technology

CPAP systems are inherently able to capture raw flow data and patterns of breathing. They currently log both raw and processed (eg, apnea-hypopnea index) information. This is currently transmitted to central data banks and it is likely that this trend will accelerate. Patients, prescribers, and insurers all have interests in various aspects of the long-term nightly CPAP signal, and the growing trend for consumer devices that provide biological data is likely to increase.

Improvements in data technology can be used to encourage patient compliance, improve treatment response, and act as warning systems. Many devices currently use Bluetooth, WiFi, and/or wireless technology to transmit daily data to cloud-based interfaces that can be used by patients, durable medical equipment providers, and clinicians. Easy availability of the raw data will enhance providers' ability to incorporate the information into clinical care.[15]

Data provided to patients can also be enhanced to improve compliance. Linking PAP data to other physiologic patient data, such as arrhythmias or glucose control, or night-time measures, such as sleep quality, by spectral analysis or actigraphy may encourage compliance. Data about body position or sleep quality could educate patients through biofeedback to improve treatment response.

Durable medical equipment companies now have access to lists of at-risk patients who have suboptimal compliance or high residual apnea-hypopnea index. Manufacturers are offering compliance management programs and services to durable medical equipment companies to try to enhance compliance in the first 90 days. Determining the optimal way to use these data is essential for improving compliance rates in the first 30 days of use, which is associated long-term compliance.

## Electronic Health Record Integration

**Box 2** lists possible benefits of linking data to the electronic medical record. Integration between vendors with cross-platform data exchange for both PAP and mandibular advancement device tracking systems would help optimize the care of patients.

If the full data sets that are collected by PAP can be exported and combined with clinical outcomes, research opportunities to learn more about sleep-disordered breathing treatment will be enhanced. Given the difficulty of performing large randomized controlled trials with PAP, this may be best way to obtain data, especially on particular patient populations. These data sets could also be used to look for novel features that may predict a good or bad response.

Automated analysis of the data especially in high-risk patients can be used to signal warning signs, such as decreases in tidal volume in obesity hypoventilation or chronic obstructive pulmonary disease patients, that may allow a provider to intervene prior to hospital admission.

## LIMITATIONS AND CHALLENGES IN IMPROVING POSITIVE AIRWAY PRESSURE TECHNOLOGY

Declining reimbursement for both diagnosis of OSA and for PAP reimbursement has the potential to reduce the investment made in PAP technological improvements. Adding to this is that PAP adherence rates have not improved much despite

---

**Box 2**
**Benefits of electronic health record linkage**

Improved provider flow/documentation

Data availability for PCP and other specialists and hospitalists

Knowledge of current settings and compliance

Linkage to other data sets for research

Automated warning systems

the technological improvements in PAP that have reached the market. Some of the potential improvements, discussed previously, may never be cost-effective for vendors to develop. Furthermore, the movement of sleep diagnostics and therapeutics out of the laboratory and into the home also may limit future research that can be obtained only with polysomnography, such as evaluating benefits of a new PAP technology on sleep structure and quality or $CO_2$ levels. Home testing, however, may also force the inclusion of more monitoring technology ($O_2$ saturation, $CO_2$ monitoring, ECG, and so forth or more advanced signals) into the PAP machines to provide continuous data.

Direct-to-consumer advertising and marketing of CPAP, which exist in some European and Australasian markets, has been extensively discussed (and maligned in the United States). If ever adopted widely in the Untied States, direct CPAP sales are likely to have a large impact on features that make the device attractive to patients as well as likely lowering the price and thus the features that can be supported in the cost-effective device.

With the advent of smaller and more portable devices, patients may purchase machines outside the insurance system. Interfacing of PAP with nonmedical device features, including smart phone control, alarm and clock functions, sound box or radio features, light therapy at end of the night, and other functions, will blur the distinction between medical and consumer uses of the PAP machine.

Finally, a major unanswered question remains as to whether any technology applied to the PAP device itself will have a significant impact on CPAP use. To date, the largest increases in reported adherence have not come from improved technology of the CPAP device but from addressing psychosocial patient issues, such as self-motivation for treatment, education, and enhancing social as well as medical support mechanisms. If this remains true, it is likely that CPAP technology will evolve less than it has in recent years, and emphasis and research efforts will focus more on patient behavior modification.

## ACKNOWLEDGMENTS

The authors thank Dr Robert Thomas for contributing his insights into the future of PAP technology and Dr Douglas Johnson for his help editorial help. We thank Stephen Marsh for information about MEMS technology and possible applications related to PAP.

## REFERENCES

1. Kenyon BJ, Reed N, Wilson A, et al, inventor; ResMed Motor Technologies Inc, assignee. Single or multiple stage blower and nested volute(s) and/or impeller(s) therefor. US patent 2017/0045056 A1. February 16, 2017.
2. Nagorny AS, Sadeghi S, Fleming DJ, et al, inventor; ResMed Motor Technologies Inc, assignee. Switch reluctance motor patent. US 2016/0336841 A1. November 17, 2016.
3. Prudlam D, Pfister PD, Richard T, inventor; MMT SA, assignee. Three-phase electric motor with a low-detent torque. US patent 9515539 B2. December 6, 2016.
4. DeVries DF Allum T, inventors; Pulmonetic Systems Inc, assignee. Mechanical ventilation system using bias valve. US Patent 2006/0249153 A1. November 9, 2006.
5. Marsh SA, inventor; Encite LLC, assignee. Micro pump systems. US patent 2015/0267695 A1. September 24, 2015.
6. Iotti G, Olivei M, Braschi A. Equipment review: mechanical effects of heat-moisture exchangers in ventilated patients. Crit Care 1999;3(5):R77–82.
7. Harrington MR, Doudkine D, Foote RML, et al, inventor; ResMed Limited, assignee. A humidifier for a respiratory therapy device. US patent 2017/0000968 A1. January 5, 2017.
8. Yilmaz B, Asyali MH, Arikan E, et al. Sleep stage and obstructive apneaic epoch classification using single-lead ECG. Biomed Eng Online 2010;9:39.
9. Thomas RJ, Mietus JE, Peng CK, et al. Differentiating obstructive from central and complex sleep apnea using an automated electrocardiogram-based method. Sleep 2007;30:1756–69.
10. SCIREQ Scientific Respiratory Equipment. Flexivent techniques and measurements. Available at: https://www.scireq.com/flexivent/techniques-and-measurements. Accessed July 31, 2017.
11. Reiter J, Zleik B, Bazalakova M, et al. Residual events during use of CPAP: prevalence, predictors, and detection accuracy. J Clin Sleep Med 2016; 12:1153–8.
12. Aurora RN, Swartz R, Punjabi NM. Misclassification of OSA severity with automated scoring of home sleep recordings. Chest 2015;147:719–27.
13. Bianchi MT, Lipoma T, Darling C, et al. Automated sleep apnea quantification based on respiratory movement. Int J Med Sci 2014;11:796–802.
14. Johnson KG, Johnson DC. Treatment of sleep-disordered breathing with positive airway pressure devices: technology update. Med Devices (Auckl) 2015;8:425–37.
15. Thomas RJ, Bianchi MT. Urgent need to improve PAP management: the devil is in two (fixable) details. J Clin Sleep Med 2017;13:657–64.

# UNITED STATES POSTAL SERVICE ®
## Statement of Ownership, Management, and Circulation (All Periodicals Publications Except Requester Publications)

| 1. Publication Title | 2. Publication Number | 3. Filing Date |
|---|---|---|
| SLEEP MEDICINE CLINICS | 025 – 053 | 9/18/2017 |

| 4. Issue Frequency | 5. Number of Issues Published Annually | 6. Annual Subscription Price |
|---|---|---|
| MAR, JUN, SEP, DEC | 4 | $203.00 |

7. Complete Mailing Address of Known Office of Publication (Not printer) (Street, city, county, state, and ZIP+4®)

ELSEVIER INC.
230 Park Avenue, Suite 800
New York, NY 10169

Contact Person
STEPHEN R. BUSHING

Telephone (Include area code)
215-239-3688

8. Complete Mailing Address of Headquarters or General Business Office of Publisher (Not printer)

ELSEVIER INC.
230 Park Avenue, Suite 800
New York, NY 10169

9. Full Names and Complete Mailing Addresses of Publisher, Editor, and Managing Editor (Do not leave blank)

Publisher (Name and complete mailing address)

ADRIANNE BRIGIDO, ELSEVIER INC.
1600 JOHN F KENNEDY BLVD. SUITE 1800
PHILADELPHIA, PA 19103-2899

Editor (Name and complete mailing address)

COLLEEN DIETZLER, ELSEVIER INC.
1600 JOHN F KENNEDY BLVD. SUITE 1800
PHILADELPHIA, PA 19103-2899

Managing Editor (Name and complete mailing address)

PATRICK MANLEY, ELSEVIER INC.
1600 JOHN F KENNEDY BLVD. SUITE 1800
PHILADELPHIA, PA 19103-2899

10. Owner (Do not leave blank. If the publication is owned by a corporation, give the name and address of the corporation immediately followed by the names and addresses of all stockholders owning or holding 1 percent or more of the total amount of stock. If not owned by a corporation, give the names and addresses of the individual owners. If owned by a partnership or other unincorporated firm, give its name and address as well as those of each individual owner. If the publication is published by a nonprofit organization, give its name and address.)

| Full Name | Complete Mailing Address |
|---|---|
| WHOLLY OWNED SUBSIDIARY OF REED/ELSEVIER, US HOLDINGS | 1600 JOHN F KENNEDY BLVD. SUITE 1800 PHILADELPHIA, PA 19103-2899 |

11. Known Bondholders, Mortgagees, and Other Security Holders Owning or Holding 1 Percent or More of Total Amount of Bonds, Mortgages, or Other Securities. If none, check box ▶ ☐ None

| Full Name | Complete Mailing Address |
|---|---|
| N/A | |

12. Tax Status (For completion by nonprofit organizations authorized to mail at nonprofit rates) (Check one)
The purpose, function, and nonprofit status of this organization and the exempt status for federal income tax purposes:
☒ Has Not Changed During Preceding 12 Months
☐ Has Changed During Preceding 12 Months (Publisher must submit explanation of change with this statement)

| 13. Publication Title | 14. Issue Date for Circulation Data Below |
|---|---|
| SLEEP MEDICINE CLINICS | JUNE 2017 |

| 15. Extent and Nature of Circulation | | Average No. Copies Each Issue During Preceding 12 Months | No. Copies of Single Issue Published Nearest to Filing Date |
|---|---|---|---|
| a. Total Number of Copies (Net press run) | | 394 | 324 |
| b. Paid Circulation (By Mail and Outside the Mail) | (1) Mailed Outside-County Paid Subscriptions Stated on PS Form 3541 (Include paid distribution above nominal rate, advertiser's proof copies, and exchange copies) | 249 | 224 |
| | (2) Mailed In-County Paid Subscriptions Stated on PS Form 3541 (Include paid distribution above nominal rate, advertiser's proof copies, and exchange copies) | 0 | 0 |
| | (3) Paid Distribution Outside the Mails Including Sales Through Dealers and Carriers, Street Vendors, Counter Sales, and Other Paid Distribution Outside USPS® | 42 | 40 |
| | (4) Paid Distribution by Other Classes of Mail Through the USPS (e.g. First-Class Mail®) | 0 | 0 |
| c. Total Paid Distribution (Sum of 15b (1), (2), (3), and (4)) ▶ | | 291 | 264 |
| d. Free or Nominal Rate Distribution (By Mail and Outside the Mail) | (1) Free or Nominal Rate Outside-County Copies included on PS Form 3541 | 58 | 60 |
| | (2) Free or Nominal Rate In-County Copies included on PS Form 3541 | 0 | 0 |
| | (3) Free or Nominal Rate Copies Mailed at Other Classes Through the USPS (e.g. First-Class Mail) | 0 | 0 |
| | (4) Free or Nominal Rate Distribution Outside the Mail (Carriers or other means) | 0 | 0 |
| e. Total Free or Nominal Rate Distribution (Sum of 15d (1), (2), (3) and (4)) ▶ | | 58 | 60 |
| f. Total Distribution (Sum of 15c and 15e) ▶ | | 349 | 324 |
| g. Copies not Distributed (See Instructions to Publishers #4 (page #3)) ▶ | | 45 | 0 |
| h. Total (Sum of 15f and g) ▶ | | 394 | 324 |
| i. Percent Paid (15c divided by 15f times 100) ▶ | | 83.38% | 81.48% |

* If you are claiming electronic copies, go to line 16 on page 3. If you are not claiming electronic copies, skip to line 17 on page 3.

| 16. Electronic Copy Circulation | Average No. Copies Each Issue During Preceding 12 Months | No. Copies of Single Issue Published Nearest to Filing Date |
|---|---|---|
| a. Paid Electronic Copies ▶ | 0 | 0 |
| b. Total Paid Print Copies (Line 15c) + Paid Electronic Copies (Line 16a) ▶ | 291 | 264 |
| c. Total Print Distribution (Line 15f) + Paid Electronic Copies (Line 16a) ▶ | 349 | 324 |
| d. Percent Paid (Both Print & Electronic Copies) (16b divided by 16c × 100) ▶ | 83.38% | 81.48% |

☒ I certify that 50% of all my distributed copies (electronic and print) are paid above a nominal price.

17. Publication of Statement of Ownership

☒ If the publication is a general publication, publication of this statement is required. Will be printed in the DECEMBER 2017 issue of this publication.

☐ Publication not required.

| 18. Signature and Title of Editor, Publisher, Business Manager, or Owner | Date |
|---|---|
| STEPHEN R. BUSHING - INVENTORY DISTRIBUTION CONTROL MANAGER | 9/18/2017 |

I certify that all information furnished on this form is true and complete. I understand that anyone who furnishes false or misleading information on this form or who omits material or information requested on the form may be subject to criminal sanctions (including fines and imprisonment) and/or civil sanctions (including civil penalties).

PS Form 3526, July 2014 (Page 1 of 4 (see instructions page 4)) PSN 7530-01-000-9931    PRIVACY NOTICE: See our privacy policy on www.usps.com.

PS Form 3526, July 2014 (Page 3 of 4)    PRIVACY NOTICE: See our privacy policy on www.usps.com

# Moving?

## Make sure your subscription moves with you!

To notify us of your new address, find your **Clinics Account Number** (located on your mailing label above your name), and contact customer service at:

**Email: journalscustomerservice-usa@elsevier.com**

**800-654-2452** (subscribers in the U.S. & Canada)
**314-447-8871** (subscribers outside of the U.S. & Canada)

**Fax number: 314-447-8029**

**Elsevier Health Sciences Division**
**Subscription Customer Service**
**3251 Riverport Lane**
**Maryland Heights, MO 63043**

*To ensure uninterrupted delivery of your subscription, please notify us at least 4 weeks in advance of move.

Printed and bound by CPI Group (UK) Ltd, Croydon, CR0 4YY

03/10/2024

01040382-0007